Gerontology and Geriatrics Libraries and Collections in the United States and Canada

Gerontology and Geriatrics Libraries and Collections in the United States and Canada

A History, Description, and Directory

JOYCE A. POST

GREENWOOD PRESS
Westport, Connecticut • London

Library of Congress Cataloging-in-Publication Data

Post, Joyce A.
Gerontology and geriatrics libraries and collections in the United States and Canada : a history, description, and directory / Joyce A. Post.
p. cm.
Includes bibliographical references and indexes.
ISBN 0-313-28443-1 (alk. paper)
1. Libraries—United States—Special collections—Aging.
2. Libraries—Canada—Special collections—Aging. 3. Libraries—Special collections—Gerontology. 4. Libraries—Special collections—Geriatrics. 5. Gerontology—Library resources.
6. Geriatrics—Library resources. 7. Old age—Library resources.
8. Aging—Library resources. 9. Aged—Library resources.
I. Title.
Z688.A58P67 1992
025.2'761267—dc20 91-46862

British Library Cataloguing in Publication Data is available.

Library of Congress Catalog Card Number: 91-46862
ISBN: 0-313-28443-1

First published in 1992

Greenwood Press, 88 Post Road West, Westport, CT 06881
An imprint of Greenwood Publishing Group, Inc.

Printed in the United States of America

The paper used in this book complies with the Permanent Paper Standard issued by the National Information Standards Organization (Z39.48-1984).

10 9 8 7 6 5 4 3 2 1

Dedicated to all
Librarians and Information Specialists
in Gerontology and Geriatrics

Past, Present, and Future

Contents

Tables

Acknowledgments

Many people contributed significantly to the success of this book. M. Powell Lawton, Director of Research at the Polisher Research Institute of the Philadelphia Geriatric Center, provided the supportive environment and encouragement as well as information about gerontology libraries in the United States in the 1940s and 1950s.

Many others at the Philadelphia Geriatric Center helped with the survey of gerontology and geriatrics libraries and collections. Mary McCaffrey, Library Assistant, made many telephone calls to obtain missing data. Loretta Steward, Data Entry, inputted all the coded data so the computer analysis could take place. Allen Glicksman, Director of Research Computer Services, gave advice on coding the data and ran the frequency distributions and cross-tabulations. Morton H. Kleban, Senior Research Psychologist, gave advice on the questionnaire design and the statistical analysis. Miriam Moss, Senior Research Sociologist, also helped with the questionnaire design and gave lots of encouragement along the way. Renee Lawrence provided information about the gerontology collection at the University of Michigan. Pat Parmelee loaned her laser printer.

Daniel J. Cragg located a copy of OMB Memorandum 81-14, "Federal Information Centers," dated September 11,

1981, that was crucial in determining the chronological sequence of events leading to the demise of the National Clearinghouse on Aging.

Maureen Neville, Librarian at the Philadelphia Corporation for Aging, the Area Agency on Aging (AAA) for Philadelphia, provided much useful information and insight about libraries at AAAs and the SCAN publications produced by the Franklin Research Center in Philadelphia.

H. Jean Owens, compiler of the 1980 Directory of Gerontological Libraries and Information Centers and Eve Rafferty, Manager of Technical Services at the American Association of Retired Persons (AARP) Research Information Center, provided valuable information about their respective surveys of gerontology and geriatrics libraries so the present findings could be compared with their results.

And finally library directors Joanna Chen Lin at the National Institute on Aging, Paula M. Lovas at the AARP Research Information Center, and Janette Hoisington at the National Council on the Aging encouraged me to proceed when this project was just a gleam in the author's eye.

Introduction

When I became a gerontology and geriatrics librarian six years ago I knew nothing about these areas of special and medical librarianship. As I grew into the position I became increasingly curious about the historical antecedents of gerontology and geriatrics libraries and collections.

I discovered that most of the writing in aging by librarians was about general library services to aging individuals, an area of library specialization quite different from special library services to the physicians, psychologists, administrators, policymakers, students, and others working in the areas of gerontology, geriatrics, and long-term care.

I also discovered that the questions I was answering covered a very wide range of disciplines. The day I was asked for a search on the adverse effects of cimetidine use in the elderly, a legislative history of a proposed amendment to the Older Americans Act (OAA), and the numbers and percentages of nursing homes discharges that are deaths was turning out to be a fairly typical day. I began to think the librarians in gerontology and geriatrics deserved a lot of respect for everything they were called upon to know.

So when an article on horticultural libraries appeared in the journal Special Libraries I decided gerontology and geriatrics libraries deserved equal attention.

Since the main library offices and the offices of most of the researchers at the Philadelphia Geriatric Center are situated in the same building wing, I was already in a supportive environment in which to carry out a survey of libraries and collections serving the professionals and students of gerontology and geriatrics. The most difficult part was finding the time to keep both the library functioning and the research ongoing.

Gerontology is the study of the aging process from maturity into old age as well as the study of the elderly as a special population. Geriatrics is the study of the medical aspects of old age. The line between these disciplines is almost never clear-cut. The physician treating an older person for hip fracture must consider whether the living arrangements of that person includes steps and stairs. The gerontologist studying depression in the elderly must be aware of the medical illnesses often accompanied by signs and symptoms of depression.

Much of the published literature in gerontology and geriatrics reflects the interdisciplinary nature of the two disciplines. This literature is quite large and most of the libraries described in this work do not attempt to build collections of equal strength in both gerontology and geriatrics. It is entirely appropriate, however, to survey gerontology and geriatrics libraries and collections in the same effort.

The present work consists of three major sections. The first is a history of gerontology and geriatrics libraries in the United States and their information activities.

The second section is a detailed and comparative analysis of the data gathered in a 1990 survey of gerontology and geriatrics libraries and collections in the United States and Canada. There were five reasons for undertaking the present research. I wanted to: (1) describe the current state of gerontology and geriatrics libraries; (2) compare the present findings with the results of three other surveys; (3) find out where the most substantial collections on aging in the United States and Canada were; (4) find out which of the collections identified in a 1980 directory of gerontology libraries were still in existence ten years later; and (5) discover and document the history and growth of gerontology and geriatrics collections and libraries and their information activities.

The third section is a directory of the 73 libraries and collections responding to the 1990 survey. It is arranged alphabetically by state, then by towns within each state, and, if necessary, alphabetically by the name of parent organization of the library or collection within each city or town.

Each library or collection has a two part code. The first part is the two-letter post office abbreviation for the state in which the library or collection is located. The one collection in Puerto Rico begins with "PR" and the five Canadian libraries begin with "CAN." The second part of the code is a consecutive number representing each library as it appears within each state section. For example, the third library/collection listed in the California section has the code CA-3, the first library/collection in Kentucky has the code KY-1, etc.

When these codes are used as finding devices in the appendices, they appear in alphabetical order according to the state represented. For example, the codes beginning with "MD" appear before those beginning with "MA" because Maryland comes before Massachusetts. The listing for Puerto Rico comes after all the state listings and the five Canadian listings follow that.

There are five appendices. Appendix A is a reproduction of the questionnaire used for the survey. Appendix B is an alphabetic list of the libraries/collections assigned to each of the eight major types of libraries/collections identified in this survey. Appendix C is a coded list of each of the 73 libraries or collections that have a current subscription to the 18 selected serial titles asked about in question IV.b. of the survey. Appendix D is a coded list of the libraries/collections that have collection strengths in each of the 21 categories used in this survey. Appendix E is a coded list of hardware and software used by those libraries/collections that specifically described their automated operations.

Questionnaires were sent to every gerontology and geriatrics library and collection that could be identified, as described in the methodology section of this book. It was difficult to assure that the questionnaire landed in the hands of the person in charge of the library or collection. No doubt some libraries and collections have been missed. In addition, some potential respondents refused to participate. I would appreciate any information about these missing collections so the omissions can be corrected in any future work.

Several new libraries and resource centers in aging have been formed since the survey was conducted. A major library on Alzheimer's disease was opened in November 1991 by The Alzheimer's Association. Patricia Pinkowski is the director of the Benjamin B. Green-Field National Alzheimer's Library and Resource Center, 919 N. Michigan Avenue, Suite 1000, Chicago, IL 60611, 312-335-9602, open Monday-Friday 8:30a.m.-5p.m. The National Institute on Aging has established an Alzheimer's Disease Education and Referral (ADEAR) Center at P.O. Box 8250, Silver Spring, MD 20907-8250, 301-495-3311. They maintain the Alzheimer's Disease subfile, an online bibliographic database that is part of the Combined Health Information Database (CHID).

A Resource Library of information on long-term care for professionals, organizations, and the general public has been established at the Orange Caregiver Resource Center at 251 East Imperial Highway, Suite 460, Fullerton, CA 92635, 714-680-0122, Joyce Bryan, Director. And ironically, almost exactly 10 years after the Administration on Aging (AoA) killed the National Clearinghouse on Aging (see pages 8-10), the AoA has announced on page 46624 of the September 13, 1991 Federal Register an internal reorganization that, among other things, promotes the establishment of an information clearinghouse to disseminate and exchange information in the field of aging.

In this time of both increasing numbers of older persons and of professionals serving them, gerontology and geriatrics libraries and librarians are resources that should be better known and supported.

The wide range of disciplines with which gerontology and geriatrics are concerned is reflected in the materials in these libraries/collections and in the knowledge of their librarians. They routinely use the information resources of medicine; psychology, social work and the other behavioral sciences; demographics, statistics, and the census; and government legislation, regulations, and policy to answer questions.

This study shows that gerontology libraries and collections are found in a wide range of parent organizations. The purpose and nature of the collections and services offered differ widely between each of the eight different types identified. There are, however, more similarities than differences and these findings are presented, not to emphasize the differences, but to celebrate the diversity.

Many of the libraries and collections are one-person libraries. Typically, the persons managing them might do everything from planning and overseeing the automation of library operations, to literature searches, to shelving new issues of journals, to charging out books, to changing the paper in various library machines. Persons working in these types of situations benefit greatly by knowing there are others out there in similar situations and that common knowledge and practical tips can be shared.

Some of the more unique aspects of librarianship and the newest ways of providing service are being practiced in some of the gerontology and geriatrics libraries and collections contributing to this work. Some of the librarians are very essential parts of various professional teams at their organization.

Some follow the principles of special librarianship and act as information managers who get the answers to the questions their clientele ask, exhibiting a more proactive "just-in-time" role than the more traditional librarian role of developing a collection "just-in-case" someone has a question and then showing them how to use that collection to find their answer.

In some of the collections described here there is a very small "home-base" collection. The information manager/librarian goes, by foot, phone, modem, or fax, to where the material is and gets what is needed. It is interesting to observe that in almost every case where these so-called innovative techniques have been adopted, it has been as an alternative to a low level of support rather than as a test of modern management techniques.

The large libraries play a very different, and very necessary, role in the overall network of gerontology and geriatrics collections. Without their extensive collections and their means to produce the reference and working tools used everyday, most of the collections described in this study would have great difficulty doing their jobs.

Gerontology and geriatrics librarians and collections seem to have been really hurt, both financially and morally, by the cutbacks in support in the early 1980s. It's time to see if some of the spirit and enthusiasm exhibited in the earlier days can be rekindled by the 23 librarians identified by this survey who said they were willing to come together and explore ways to be more interconnected.

It is my hope that this work contributes to an understanding of the historical background and current state of gerontology and geriatrics libraries and collections.

Gerontology and Geriatrics Libraries and Collections in the United States and Canada

1

History and Information Activities in the United States

The discipline of gerontology in the United States began in 1939 and within the next decade activities had gained momentum on several different fronts. In 1939 the first edition of E. V. Cowdry's Problems of Ageing, the first definitive modern compilation of what was known about aging at the time, was published. Also in that year the Club for Research on Ageing was organized and became the Gerontological Society in 1945 and the Gerontological Society of America (GSA) in 1980 (Achenbaum, 1987; Adler, 1958). GSA's first journal, the Journal of Gerontology, began publication in 1946. In 1940 the first major research effort in gerontology began and in the 1950s several university programs in the field were established.

The importance of bibliographic activities and library collections in gerontology was recognized from the beginning and this section is a look at these activities.

ORIGINAL BIBLIOGRAPHIC ACTIVITIES

The first library-type activity in gerontology began with the publication in 1951 of Nathan W. Shock's A Classified Bibliography of Gerontology and Geriatrics listing all publications pertinent to gerontology known at that time. It was kept current with supplements published in 1957 (Shock, 1957) and 1963 (Shock, 1963) and by Shock's classified listings in the "Index to Current Periodical Literature" column in each issue of the Journal of Gerontology published between April 1950 and November 1980. It was suspended at that time because the gerontology literature had grown quite large and an automated method of bibliographic control of aging materials was in the planning stage (Shock, 1982).

EARLIEST LIBRARY COLLECTIONS

One of the earliest gerontology collections was developed to support the Baltimore Longitudinal Study of Aging (BLSA) begun in 1958 at the Gerontology Research Center (GRC) at the Baltimore City Hospitals. The BLSA (Shock, et al., 1984, pp. 45-46; 1987) was an expansion of an earlier program begun in 1940 at the GRC. From the beginning the GRC had operated within the administrative framework of the National Institutes of Health and when the National Institute on Aging (NIA) was established in 1974 all GRC research activities, including the BLSA and the gerontology collection, were transferred to NIA (Butler, 1987). The collection formed the basis for the present Gerontology Resource Center Library of the National Institute on Aging located on the former grounds of the Baltimore City Hospitals at the present Francis Scott Key Medical Center in Baltimore.

During the 1950s and 1960s several gerontology collections were developed at universities where there were strong research and professional education programs. Two of the oldest of these programs still in existence today are the Scripps Gerontology Center at Miami University in Oxford, Ohio, founded in 1922 as a center for population studies, and the Center for Gerontological Studies at the University of Florida in Gainesville, founded in 1951. Both presently maintain small office collections of books and current journals designed to serve their faculty and research staff but are without the management services of a professional librarian.

The first major university gerontology library was established in 1965 at the Institute of Gerontology at the University of Michigan in Ann Arbor. During the 1970s it joined forces with Wayne State University in Detroit and together they became a major U. S. library of aging materials. In the early

1980s a new director came to the Institute—a biochemist, who wanted the library space, which consisted of an open-stack reading room with seating for 16 people, a separate audiovisual room, and a librarians' office, for laboratories. Nearly all the books were transferred to the University of Michigan medical library in 1986. All the historical papers went to the University archives. The bound journals and some of Nathan W. Shock's books have been kept at the Institute in the Wilma Donahue/Nathan Shock Library which is now basically a "frozen-in-time" office collection (W. Andrew Achenbaum, personal communication, July 28, 1991).

The experience of the Andrus Gerontology Center Library at the University of Southern California in Los Angeles and begun in 1966 is typical of how most of the early collections grew. It began as an office collection of 150 books and four journals located in the executive director's office and was used by students in the program (*Catalogs of the Ethel Percy Andrus Gerontology Center*, 1976, vol. 1, pp. iii; Longo, Greathouse, and Mueller, 1982). It is now the only major separate gerontology library in the United States located at a university.

The oldest gerontology/geriatrics libraries affiliated with medical/nursing home facilities were established at the Jewish Home and Hospital for the Aged in New York City in 1942, at the Philadelphia Geriatric Center in 1959, and at the Maimonides Hospital Geriatric Centre in Montreal, Canada, in 1965. All three libraries are still in existence and all offer a full range of library services including extensive collections in geriatrics which the largest gerontology libraries do not have.

The libraries at gerontology associations are among the oldest and largest in both the United States and Canada. The oldest one in the United States, begun in 1950, is at the National Council on the Aging in Washington, D.C. In addition to being the second largest gerontology library in the United States, it produces the quarterly <u>Abstracts in Social Gerontol-</u>

ogy (formerly Current Literature on Aging).

The American Association of Retired Persons (AARP) Research Information Center, also in Washington, D.C., began in 1965 and grew out of the earlier collections of the National Retired Teachers Association (NRTA) and AARP. It is the largest gerontology library in the United States and is the producer of the AgeLine database. From 1965 to October 1991 the name of this library was the National Gerontology Resource Center.

Until 1990, the oldest geriatrics/gerontology library in Canada was the J. W. Crane Library of Geriatrics and Gerontology sponsored by the Canadian Geriatrics Research Society and located in a municipal home for the aged in Toronto (Duwors, Marshall, and Moore, 1982; Grant, 1986). It was established in 1962. In 1990 it merged with the Deer Lodge Resource Centre in Gerontology and Geriatrics in Winnipeg. The merged collection, now the largest geriatrics and gerontology collection in Canada, retains the original name of the J. W. Crane Memorial Library but is housed at the Winnipeg location in Manitoba.

Those libraries from this original group that endure today do so because of the trustworthy support of their parent bodies and the continuing vision of their directors who have seen them through periods of fluctuating financial support for gerontology research and independence from close scrutiny of their programs by grant-issuing agencies.

UNITED STATES FEDERAL INVOLVEMENT

Other collections of gerontology and geriatrics resources and at least one of the major information activities in the field were created by government programs. The fortunes of many of these have been tied directly to this support which has been called capricious by some.

The major piece of legislation for this support is the Older Americans Act of 1965 (OAA) (Ficke, 1985) which established the Administration on Aging (AoA) within the then Office of the Secretary of Health, Education, and Welfare.

The Second White House Conference on Aging took place in 1971 and its recommendations are thought to have directly influenced the far-reaching effects of the 1973 amendments to the OAA. One of the mandates of these amendments was the creation of the State Units on Aging (SUA) and the Area Agencies on Aging (AAA) hierarchy. Each SUA is responsible for developing an overall plan for the provision of services for the elderly within its state and each AAA acts as the coordinator of all the services for the elderly within its geographic area. At the present time there are 50 individual SUAs and over 650 local AAAs. This federal-state-local network, AoA-SUA-AAA, is collectively known as the aging network and is the provider of such programs for aging individuals as Meals on Wheels, information and referral services, access to transportation, housing assistance, and ombudsman activities (Gelfand, 1988; Oriol, 1987).

The oldest of the SUA/AAA gerontology libraries began in state departments of aging before the original OAA was enacted. The oldest known and still existing libraries in SUAs were established in 1958 at the Rhode Island Department of Elderly Affairs in Providence and at the Tennessee Commission on Aging in Nashville in 1963. When the State Units on Aging hierarchy was created in 1973 by the OAA, these already existing agencies moved into this new role.

The same pattern is true for two of the seven identified Area Agencies on Aging with libraries. The New York City Department of Aging Library began in 1970 and the City of Chicago Department on Aging and Disability Library began in 1972. The other five AAA libraries were established between 1974 and 1980.

The existence of collections and libraries in SUAs/AAAs

has been directly related to the political thinking and funding of aging policies in vogue at any given time. Those that have endured have done so because someone at each agency was of the very firm belief that a collection or library was necessary and saw to it that this belief did not waver over time.

From the beginning the OAA authorized appropriations for multidisciplinary centers of gerontology (MCG) at institutions of higher learning. This led to the establishment of the Association for Gerontology in Higher Education in 1972 (Hickey, 1978) and specific appropriations to fund MCGs in fiscal years 1976 through 1980 (Ficke, 1985, pp. 37-40; Simson and Wilson, 1981). However, with the 1981 amendments to the OAA, all support for education/training and research was consolidated into discretionary funds (Craig, 1982; Peterson and Douglass, 1990). The idea to fund the MCGs grew out of the success of the original university gerontology programs started in the 1940s and 1950s prior to the enactment of the OAA. Under the MCG program many additional academic gerontology programs were started and some of them developed their own library collections. The establishment of gerontology collections of this type peaked between 1975 and 1978 and ceased after 1982.

NATIONAL CLEARINGHOUSE ON AGING/SERVICE CENTER FOR AGING INFORMATION

The 1973 amendments to the OAA authorized the establishment of a National Information and Resource Clearinghouse for Aging. Money was appropriated for the Clearinghouse for fiscal years 1978 through 1982. In addition to the more traditional clearinghouse functions of providing public information and statistical analysis, the Clearinghouse also planned to take on responsibility for the development of a system of bibliographic control of aging literature and material, much of which is of a fugitive report nature and difficult to locate. The idea of federally supported human services information clearinghouses was popular at this time (Applied Management Sciences, and Cuadra Associates, 1980, 1981; Baker and Bale, 1981) and planning for the bibliographic activities of the National Clearinghouse on Aging began in 1975 (United States. Congress. Senate. Special Committee on Aging, 1974, p. 104; 1975, pp. 188-191; 1976, pp. 70-75; 1977, pp. 73-74, 83-84; 1978, pp. 54, 62-63; 1979, pp. 96-97). By 1980 several phases of this part of the program had been implemented including a Service Center for Aging Information (SCAN) to administer the collection, announcement, and dissemination activities of the bibliographic effort (Smith, 1983; United States. Congress. Senate. Special Committee on Aging, 1980, p. 85; 1981, p. 99) and the first two editions of a thesaurus of aging terminology for use by the SCAN system (United States. Administration on Aging. National Clearinghouse on Aging, 1975, 1977).

Encouraged by this funding for education in gerontology and the National Clearinghouse on Aging, a discernable beginning in interest in resource sharing and networking activities can be seen by the librarians of the major gerontology and geriatrics collections in existence at that time. They started writing (Ardito and Dosa, 1983; Bagnell, 1982; Dosa, 1978; Miller and Cutler, 1976; Rafferty, 1982; United States. General Accounting Office, 1976; Van Steenberg and Karasik, 1978; Wanted: Information about and for the aging, 1978; Zito, Miller, and Herrera, 1985) and presenting papers (Brindle, Dosa, and Gee, 1977; Corcoran, 1982; Dosa and Brindle, 1979; Gilbert, 1981; Rafferty and Dosa, 1980; Shock, Dosa, Monroe, Edwards, and Flynn, 1977) about collection development and information sharing. In addition, two surveys of existing collections were made (Owens, 1978; Rafferty, 1983), and a directory of gerontology collections was compiled (Owens, 1980).

Almost immediately after Ronald Reagan was installed as President in January 1981, it became evident that the 1981 amendments to the OAA were going to eliminate much of the earlier funding and programs. In the cases of the National Clearinghouse on Aging and SCAN the cuts were swift and total. As early as February 25, 1981 the Office of Management and Budget (OMB) stated its intention to cut funding for the Clearinghouse (Reagan deferrals could mean big loss to senior centers, 1981; Reagan signs recissions bill, 1981, p. 2). By June 10th funding was "zeroed-out" of both the Senate and House OAA authorization bills (Democrats plan new strategy for OAA programs, 1981, p. 2; House Republican move could cost OAA millions, 1981, p. 4). On September 11th, in accordance with the directives of the Paperwork Reduction Act of 1980, OMB issued Memorandum 81-14 questioning the government's support of Federal Information Centers and requiring the heads of executive departments and agencies to evaluate their information activities and implement information resources management (United States. Executive Office of the President. Office of Management and Budget, 1981). When the 1981 OAA amendments and authorizations were signed into law on December 29, 1981, the Clearinghouse was eliminated (United States. Congress. Senate. Special Committee on Aging, 1982, p. 389).

Although it took a while for the impact of these directives and cuts to be felt, it was with the 1981 OAA amendments that the Reagan administration made one of its first and most clear-cut impacts in government policies on aging (Achenbaum, 1983, chapter 6) and information (Hernon and McClure, 1987, chapter 7; Larson and Ruhl, 1981).

SCAN activities had grown slowly between 1977 and early 1981. The system was designed to be similar to the Educational Resources Information Center (ERIC) with a Central Control Facility and two Resource Centers, one for biomedicine and one for social gerontology. Early contracts to operate the facility and centers were awarded between 1978 and 1980 (First SCAN contract awarded, 1978) but were less than successful. Some things were accomplished during this period, however. In 1979 a set of approximately 3,000 source documents in aging published as far back as 1966 and comprising mostly the final reports of projects funded by AoA had been microfiched and placed at over 230 sites, mostly at universities, around the United States (*Subject index to the SCAN microfiche collection*, 1987). Two of the publications issued in October 1980 by the Social Behavioral Science Resource Center at the Franklin Research Center in Philadelphia are typical of what was hoped for through the SCAN system (*Aging and long-term care*, 1980; *A guide to selected information resources in aging*, 1980).

Ironically, it was in 1981 that SCAN activities began to gather momentum. In January 1981 a contract was awarded for the Central Control Facility and by April 1981 descriptive cataloging of the documents in the collection began. By February 1982 separate bibliographies were available on 78 different topics, by March 1982 the SCAN bibliographic database became accessible online through BRS, by June 1982 more than 12,000 documents were in various stages of processing, and by September 1982 all SCAN services to the public were terminated.

The Administration on Aging recognized the value of the SCAN database and solicited proposals for the assumption of its bibliographic activities. The successful applicant (Halpin, 1985) was the library at AARP which had became the National Gerontology Resource Center (Lovas, 1982) and is now the AARP Research Information Center. The original SCAN database was the foundation from which the current AgeLine database was created and the thesaurus for this database is the original thesaurus created for SCAN and is now in its fourth edition (*Thesaurus of aging terminology*, 1991).

GERIATRIC EDUCATION CENTERS

Professionals in aging usually concentrate their interests and work in either the behavioral or medical aspects of the field. Much of the financial support for education and training in the behavioral, or gerontological, aspects has been through the Administration on Aging's previously described multidisciplinary centers of gerontology and subsequent discretionary funding. Financial support for education and training in the medical, or geriatric, aspects has not been around as long.

In 1983 the Health Resources and Services Administration of the U.S. Public Health Service began funding Geriatric Education Centers (GEC) to "facilitate training of faculty, students and practitioners in medicine, dentistry, optometry, pharmacy, podiatric medicine, nursing, and appropriate allied and public health disciplines in the diagnosis, treatment, and prevention of diseases and other health problems of the aged . . . . These Centers emphasize faculty and curriculum development, consultation, information dissemination, technical assistance, and continuing education . . . . " (*Geriatric education centers*, 1989, preface).

In 1989 there were 39 GECs in the United States and Puerto Rico. The major affiliation of all of them is with one or more local university medical schools and/or medical centers. Many, however, also have strong cooperative working arrangements with gerontology centers that are at the same universities. For example, the Pacific Geriatric Education Center at the University of Southern California (USC) School of Medicine draws direct support of a nonfinancial nature from the Andrus Gerontology Center, also at USC. At the Duke University GEC the Director is also the Director of the Duke University Center for the Study of Aging and Human Development. And the U. M. Pomerance Library and Resource Center at the University of Miami School of Medicine serves both the Center for Adult Development and Aging at the University of Miami and the Miami Area Geriatric Education Center at the university medical school.

There is a wide variety in the ways individual GECs carry out their mission (Hubbard and Kowal, 1988), but almost all of them offer an information/resource-sharing component. This, too, varies widely. Some provide on-the-spot cataloged educational resource centers (the word library is not used); some provide the services of an experienced database searcher who uses the university library to do searches and locate materials for GEC participants; some provide listings of regional library resources in gerontology and geriatrics; some provide seminars on information resources in aging.

NATIONAL AGING RESOURCE CENTERS

In fiscal year 1988 the AoA authorized the establishment of 11 National Aging Resource Centers to be funded for a three-year period (New National Aging Resource Centers, 1989; United States. Congress. Senate. Special Committee on Aging, 1991, p. 187-198.) Each has responsibility for a specific aspect of long-term care and each is to collect information on successful models of service delivery to aging individuals for use by the aging network. All are located at already existing university gerontology centers or aging organizations.

As the three-year-funding period for the resource centers was about to expire, AoA announced new funding for 13 National Eldercare Institutes to take their place, each also concentrating on a specific aspect of long-term care (Abortion issue puts veto threat on FY'92 funding for AoA, 1991; Applications due June 28 for AoA eldercare institutes, 1991). These latest examples illustrate how difficult it is for gerontology centers and aging organizations to engage in long-range planning. Many are largely dependent on AoA funding and yet the unpredictability of this funding over time in supporting aging programs seems to guarantee that much of it is wasteful. AoA-supported programs have little time to examine the good and bad points of existing programs before they must retrench to capture a piece of the newest round of government funding.

This unpredicability of AoA funding is directly reflected in the amount of library and information service available at individual university gerontology centers and aging organizations. Higher levels of these services are usually found where a large part of the activity is supported by funds for aging research from the National Institute on Aging, the National Institute of Mental Health, and private sources rather than for programs supported by AoA funding.

However much the intensity of library and information services provided at each location varies, this service almost never gets beyond day-to-day service to the practitioners at the parent organization. Gerontology and geriatrics librarians have met occasionally since 1981 to share collection strengths and ideas for resource sharing but have not been able to develop any specific cooperative or long-range plans in these areas.

Although no one denies the rising numbers and percentages of older people and the need to better understand the behavioral and clinical aspects of aging, the federal government has not had any clearly understood, nonfragmenated, sustained directives in aging (Jacobs, 1990) and in the provision of aging services (United States. Congress. Office of Technology Assessment, 1990). Federal aging policies and federal information policies have both directly influenced the depth and breadth of library and information services activities presently available in gerontology. One specific example of this impact is that librarians in gerontology and geriatrics have published nothing and done very little networking since those bibliographically optimistic days of the early 1980s.

2

Description of Collections in the United States and Canada

Despite the setbacks in library and information services in gerontology and geriatrics in the 1980s, it was evident that significant libraries and collections in these subject areas existed in 1990. In addition, it was now at least ten years since the first survey (Owens, 1978) and directory (Owens, 1980) of gerontology and geriatrics libraries and collections had been published. The time seemed right for a new survey and directory and work began toward that end early in 1990.

METHODOLOGY

The questionnaire was developed in the first quarter of 1990 using many of the questions from the 1989 American Hospital Association (AHA) Survey of Health Sciences Libraries in Hospitals (American Hospital Association, 1990). While searching for a group of general survey questions that could be used to describe a special library, the investigator received the AHA questionnaire. Parts of it seemed appropriate for the present effort and there was the additional bonus that the results of the two surveys could be compared. Most of the AHA libraries and the gerontology and geriatrics libraries to be surveyed were known to be small and therefore hopefully to have similar bases for comparison. The investigator also included questions in the final questionnaire so that results could be compared with the findings of the two known previous surveys of gerontology and geriatrics libraries (Owens, 1978; Rafferty, 1983). See Appendix A for the questionnaire used for this survey.

Names of potential respondents were taken from five sources: the latest editions of the Directory of Special Libraries and Information Centers (Darnay and DeMaggio, 1990) and the Research Centers Directory (Dresser and Hill, 1990), the 1980 Directory of Gerontological Libraries and Information Centers (Owens, 1980), the 1989 descriptive list of Geriatric Education Centers (*Geriatric education centers*, 1989), and a descriptive list of the National Aging Resource Centers (New National Aging Resource Centers, 1989).

In the spring of 1990 questionnaires were mailed to 157 collections and libraries—149 in the United States and 8 in Canada. Of these, 109 were returned and an additional 19 were interviewed over the telephone in the fall of 1990 using an abbreviated version of the questionnaire for a response rate of 80 percent. Five potential respondents refused to answer the questionnaire no matter how often the value of their response was explained or how many messages were left to return our telephone calls.

Of the returned questionnaires, 55 responses were not considered appropriate for inclusion in the analysis. Eight were returned unanswered saying their collection was too small; 14 said the collection had been merged into a larger, more general collection; and 9 said the collection was no longer maintained or functioning. The rest were not used because there was no evidence of a collection with a gerontology or geriatrics emphasis. Many of the 55 responses not used were from collections that had lost support because of the Reagan administration cutbacks described in Part I.

The data were analyzed using the BMDP-PC statistical software package (*BMDP data manager*, 1990) on a Novell network. Frequency distributions were computed for all 271 variables. Cross tabulations were completed for selected variables by eight different types of library/collections. The variables chosen for cross tabulation by library type were thought to be indicators of dynamic library service: presence of at least one full-time professional librarian, number of monograph titles held, number of journal titles currently received, number of reference questions answered and number of books circulated in a month, number of interlibrary loans received and sent in a month, and evidence of a diverse clientele.

RESULTS

Geographic Location

Of the 73 responses used for this survey, 40 percent were from collections located in the northeastern part of the United States, 22 percent were in the Midwest, 18 percent were in the West, and 12 percent were in the South. Five libraries, or 7 percent, were in Canada and one library was in Puerto Rico.

Types of Libraries and Collections

The libraries and collections fall into eight distinct types when their parent organizations, the nature of their collections, and the services they provide are examined. Table 1 shows the distribution of the different types. Appendix B lists each library/collection by type.

Many of the original gerontology collections began with the support of academic institutions, as described in Part I, and it is clear that many of the present gerontology collections also exist with this same support. Some of the original separate collections have been integrated into their main university library, as has happened with most of the original library at the Institute of Gerontology at the University of Michigan-Wayne State University. The oldest of the original university libraries still existing as a major separate collection is at the Andrus Gerontology Center at the University of Southern California.

Many of the present separate university gerontology center collections serve largely as resource centers for students rather than as more traditional special libraries or collections. Others serve as private collections for groups of biomedical and physiology researchers studying the effects of aging.

Table 1
Types of Collections (n = 73)

Academic institutions[1]	19(26%)
Hospitals, nursing homes, university medical centers with service orientation	14(19%)
State Units on Aging/Area Agencies on Aging (SUA/AAA)	13(18%)
Associations	9(12%)
Geriatric Education Centers (GEC)	8(11%)
Research centers (nonacademic); private, nonprofit organizations	4(6%)
Government (federal, state, local) (except AAAs)	3(4%)
National Resource Centers (NRC)	3(4%)

[1]Many academic institutions also function as Geriatric Education Centers and National Resource Centers.

Whatever their focus, all collections housed at academic institutions are examined as a single group since their primary raison d'etre is to support the study and research of the staff and students at their gerontology center.

The clinical aspects of aging are of more recent interest as evidenced by the growing numbers of books and journals published on geriatric topics, physicians specializing in geriatric medicine, and nursing and allied health staff caring for aging individuals. Libraries serving this clinical interest, as opposed to those serving biomedical research in aging, form the second largest category, 19 percent, of collections studied for this survey. Of all the types of libraries/collections examined by the present survey, the ones at medical facilities and nursing homes seem to have had the least problems with continuous and reliable support from their parent organizations and seem to have been fairly immune to the uncertainties of government funding in aging.

Libraries at Area Agencies on Aging (AAA) are a very unique category of collections. They exist mainly to serve the personnel at their organizations who are often very interested in program planning and evaluation. These libraries count as their clientele the practitioners and service providers who are providing community services to aging individuals and are often the most publicly visible of all the libraries examined for this study. Strictly speaking, AAA libraries are government libraries, but their mission is so different from other types of government libraries, which exhibit more similarities than differences even though the levels of government from which they spring are different, that it is useful to examine these as two separate groups.

Seven AAAs with libraries were identified by the present study. They are in Chicago, New York City, Philadelphia, Tucson (Pima County), Arizona, and three are located in Michigan in Detroit, Grand Rapids, and Southfield. The State Units on Aging (SUA) operate in a planning, rather than service environment, and the present study identified six SUA libraries. They are located in the state capitals of Delaware, Minnesota, Ohio, Rhode Island, Tennessee, and Texas. In the small states of Delaware and Rhode Island the SUA and the one AAA in the state have a common office. Most AAA and SUA collections are small and those that are not managed by a professional librarian are tended most often by a person with the title of program specialist.

The specific categories of Geriatric Education Centers (GEC) and National Resource Centers (NRC) used in this survey are for those not affiliated with an already existing academic gerontology center. The replies of more than eight GECs have been counted here because several are at universities and are included in the numbers for that library/collection type. In many cases it is difficult to trace those original university gerontology centers and their collections established in the 1970s as they evolved through subsequent transitions to GECs between 1983 and 1987 and to NRCs in the very late 1980s.

Often the distinctions between the types of libraries/collections identified by the present survey are fuzzy. The Philadelphia Geriatric Center Library, for example, is located in a medical/nursing home facility and has an extensive geriatrics collection for its full-time medical staff and fellows, but the largest part of its collection is devoted to gerontological material used heavily by its large full-time behavioral research staff and Ph.D. candidates at local universities with programs in gerontology. In cases like this, for the analysis of the data collected by this survey, a collection is coded according to the nature of its parent organization.

Until now, these widely differing types of gerontology and geriatrics libraries and collections have not been fully recognized. The two previous surveys of gerontology libraries did recognize different types. Owens (1978) describes three different categories: gerontology libraries/learning resources centers, special/private collections, and general university library collections. Rafferty (1983, pp. 9, 12) makes distinctions between four categories: academic, aging organizations, government, and "other" libraries.

Hours, Space and Seating

Seventy-six percent of the libraries are staffed 40 hours a week during regular business hours, 6 percent are staffed more than that, and 15 percent are staffed less than that. Three percent didn't answer the question. Owens (1978) found that her 46 libraries averaged 40 hours a week. The 1989 AHA survey of 2,167 hospital libraries (American Hospital Association [AHA], 1991, p. 9) found that more than 70

Table 2
Facility Size (n = 73)

AREA	
Less than 300 square feet	30(41%)
300-1,000 square feet	19(26%)
More than 1,000 square feet	10(14%)
No answer	14(19%)
SEATING	
1-5 seats	25(34%)
6 or more seats	39(53%)
No seats	5(7%)
No answer	4(6%)

percent were staffed for at least 40 hours a week.

Table 2 shows, for the gerontology libraries/collections, the size of the library area in square feet and the number of seats provided. Comments added to the questionnaires received from the SUAs/AAAs, the GECs, the NRCs, and the association libraries, 45 percent of the total, indicate these often are not separate, dedicated library areas. Many are housed in areas also serving as meeting rooms and/or offices, with use of the book collection and equipment shared by both office staff and collection users. Often the collection is housed in bookcases lining the walls of these areas; in one case, the "library" was one wall in a 40 seat classroom.

In comparing seating and area it is interesting to observe that the highest numbers are in more seating and smaller area. One wonders how all those seats are squeezed into the square footage given for the same collection! The AHA survey (1991, p. 5) found that 50 percent of their respondents reported 1,083 square feet or less. Ten seats was the most frequently given seating capacity.

Staff

Table 3 describes the overall staffing patterns of the libraries/collections in the present survey. Just under half, 49 percent, have a professional librarian. Of those with librarians, 21 libraries, or 60 percent, have one full-time librarian and two libraries, or 6 percent, have more than one full-time librarian. Table 4 shows where the librarians are by library type. The academic and medical facilities had the highest percentages of at least one full-time librarian, the association and government libraries were the only types having more than one full-time librarian, and none of the GECs and NRCs had professional librarians.

Owens (1978) found that 67 percent of her libraries had professional librarians and thought this number was surprisingly high. The AHA survey (1991, p. 7) found that 85 percent of the libraries surveyed had professional staff, and of these, 70 percent had at least one full-time professional staff.

The "person-in-charge" of 33 percent of the libraries/collections in the present survey is called the librarian, library technician, library consultant, etc. In 7 percent of the collections they are called the information manager, information specialist, information officer, etc. The true nature of 53 percent of the collections is revealed by the wide variety of other titles of the person-in-charge: director of the center, research analyst, administrative assistant, director of medical records, coordinator of programs and publications, training officer, professor, director of communications, chief of public relations, community education supervisor, program specialist, department secretary, etc.

The highest degree obtained by 48 percent of the persons-in-charge is a library or information science degree or certificate. Twenty-three percent have a master's or Ph.D. degree in another discipline, 22 percent have a bachelor's degree, and 3 percent have an associate degree.

Table 3
Staff[1,2] (n = 71)

Type	1 (% having staff)	More than 1[3] (% having staff)	None (% of total sample)
LIBRARIANS[4]			36(51%)
full-time	21(60%)	2(6%)	
part-time	13(37%)	1(3%)	
PARAPROFESSIONALS			32(45%)
full-time	7(18%)	1(3%)	
part-time	24(62%)	7(18%)	
STUDENTS/ASSISTANTS			40(56%)
full-time	3(10%)	1(3%)	
part-time	18(58%)	9(29%)	
VOLUNTEERS			61(86%)
full-time	0	0	
part-time	6(60%)	5(50%)	

1 Respondents may have both full time and part time staff within any type.
2 Two respondents (3%) didn't answer the question.
3 Figures represent number of collections, not number of staff.
4 With professional library degree or certificate.

Table 4

Full-Time Professional Librarians by Type of Collection[1,2] (n = 23)

Type (number of cases)	1 (% with full time librarians)	More than 1 (% with full time librarians)	None (% of type)
Academic (19)	6(26%)	0	12(63%)
Medical (14)	7(30%)	0	7(50%)
SUAs/AAAs (13)	3(13%)	0	9(69%)
Associations (9)	2(9%)	1(4%)	6(67%)
GECs (8)	0	0	8(100%)
Research (4)	2(9%)	0	2(50%)
Government (3)	1(4%)	1(4%)	1(33%)
NRCs (3)	0	0	3(100%)

[1]Two respondents (3%) didn't answer the question.
[2]Percentages may not equal 100 due to rounding.

Forty-one percent of the persons-in-charge have been in that position more than four years, 29 percent have held the position less than two years, and 26 percent have held the position for two to four years.

Equipment

Seventy-three percent of the libraries surveyed had, or had access to, a photocopy machine; 51 percent had, or had access to, a microcomputer; 44 percent had audiovisual equipment; 36 percent had, or had access to, telefacsimile equipment; 22 percent had a micrographics reader or reader/printer; 12 percent had access to a minicomputer; 8 percent had access to a mainframe computer; and 4 percent had CD-ROM equipment. The AHA survey (1991, p. 5) results are approximately the same, with the following ranking of specific equipment types in decreasing order of frequency: photocopy machine, audiovisual equipment, telefacsimile machine, microcomputer, reader/printer, mainframe computer, CD-ROM player, and minicomputer.

The libraries in the gerontology survey don't anticipate much in the way of future purchases. Six percent said they were considering a CD-ROM player, 4 percent indicated the eventual purchase of a microcomputer, and 1 percent said they might be getting either a fax machine or audiovisual equipment.

Collections

Table 5 shows the types of materials in the libraries and collections responding to the questionnaire. Most of them are small in the numbers of monograph titles held and serials currently received.

Table 5
Collection Holdings[1] (n = 73)

Materials	Number (% of responses)	None (% of responses)	No answer (% of total sample)
MONOGRAPHS		5(8%)	11(15%)
500 or less	22(35%)		
501-2,000	16(26%)		
2,001-6,000	12(19%)		
More than 6,000	7(11%)		
SERIALS[2]		7(10%)	2(3%)
1-25	34(48%)		
26-100	16(23%)		
More than 100	14(20%)		
VIDEOCASSETTES	42(69%)	19(31%)	12(16%)
AUDIOCASSETTES	26(43%)	34(57%)	13(18%)
MICROFILM/FICHE	10(18%)	45(82%)	18(25%)
CD-ROM	3(6%)	50(94%)	20(27%)
PAMPHLET FILE	44(73%)	16(27%)	13(18%)
SPECIAL COLLECTIONS	15(26%)	43(74%)	15(21%)

[1]Percentages may not equal 100 due to rounding.
[2]Currently received.

Compared to the present survey, which found that 61 percent of the collections had 2,000 or fewer monograph titles and 80 percent had 6,000 or fewer monograph titles, Owens (1978) found the average size of her gerontology library/learning resources centers was 2,000 volumes and Rafferty (1983) found that 62 percent had less than 5,000 volumes. The findings of the present study more closely resemble those of the AHA survey (1991, p. 7) which found that 50 percent had fewer than 1,200 titles and 75 percent had 3,000 or fewer titles. The AHA totals, however, include both book and periodical titles. Some caution is advised in this last comparison because the scope of gerontology is wider than for clinical medicine and gerontology libraries as a whole tend to have a wider universe of monographs than the average hospital library. The collections with the biggest numbers of audiovisual material are found in SUAs/AAAs, GECs, and NRCs, a finding consistent with most of these types of collections' perceptions of themselves as learning resource centers rather than libraries.

Comments attached to the returned questionnaires of many of the smaller collections in the present survey seem to indicate a minimal amount of attention is given to the development and/or maintenance of these collections. This is often not by choice, but rather because the person responsible for the library has additional responsibilities. Some did not know how many monograph titles were in their collection; in some, unbound uncataloged report material forms the largest part of the collection; in others, there are very large numbers of file drawers housing reprint collections and reports. Much of the essential literature of gerontology is indeed of a report nature requiring some sort of cataloging if it is to be made accessible to users. This is a luxury many of the small collections do not seem to have.

Tables 6 and 7 show which types of collections have the largest and smallest numbers of monographs and serials cur-

Table 6
Number of Monographs by Type of Collection[1,2] (n = 57)

Type (number of cases)	-501 (% with monographs)	501-2,000 (% with monographs)	2,001-6,000 (% with monographs)	6,001+ (% with monographs)	None (% of type)
Academic (19)	8(14%)	2(4%)	3(5%)	1(2%)	1(5%)
Medical (14)	4(7%)	5(9%)	3(5%)	1(2%)	0
SUAs/AAAs (13)	4(7%)	3(5%)	3(5%)	0	1(8%)
Associations (9)	1(2%)	2(4%)	2(4%)	2(4%)	0
GECs (8)	3(5%)	2(4%)	0	0	2(25%)
Research (4)	1(2%)	1(2%)	0	1(2%)	1(25%)
Government (3)	0	0	1(2%)	2(4%)	0
NRCs (3)	1(2%)	1(2%)	0	0	0

[1]Eleven respondents (15%) didn't answer the question.
[2]Percentages may not equal 100 due to rounding.

Table 7

Number of Currently Received Serials by Type of Collection[1,2] (n = 64)

Type (number of cases)	1-25 (% with serials)	26-100 (% with serials)	101+ (% with serials)	None (% of type)
Academic (19)	11(17%)	4(6%)	1(2%)	3(16%)
Medical (14)	5(8%)	3(5%)	5(8%)	0
SUAs/AAAs (13)	9(14%)	3(5%)	1(2%)	0
Associations (9)	4(6%)	2(3%)	3(5%)	0
GECs (8)	4(6%)	1(2%)	0	3(38%)
Research (4)	0	1(2%)	2(3%)	1(25%)
Government (3)	0	1(2%)	2(3%)	0
NRCs (3)	1(2%)	1(2%)	0	0

[1] Two respondents (3%) didn't answer the question.

[2] Percentages may not equal 100 due to rounding.

rently received. Five libraries said they had no monographs and seven said they had no currently received serials. When these figures are looked at in conjunction with the lowest ranges of numbers of holdings for monographs and serials, it becomes apparent that many of the collections in academic facilities are small. This is a surprising finding and somewhat difficult to interpret. It may be that academic gerontology centers rely heavily on their main university libraries for most materials and keep only the very specialized and most heavily used materials in the center collection.

The types of the largest collections, on the other hand, are not unexpected.

Special Collections

Eleven of the libraries responding to this survey described their special, historical, and/or archival collections. The Andrus Gerontology Library at the University of Southern California in Los Angeles has a copy of the SCAN microfiche collection produced by the National Clearinghouse on Aging in 1979 and a collection of papers by and about Ethel Percy Andrus. The AARP Research Information Center has two extensive collections: background materials used for the 1971 and 1981 White House Conferences on Aging and the hearings and reports of the House and Senate Special Committees on Aging. The National Council on the Aging Library has the papers of Ollie A. Randall. The Library at the National Institute on Aging has the papers relating to the early bibliographies published by Nathan W. Shock and many of the monographs of early gerontological researchers. The Jewish Home and Hospital for the Aged Library in New York City has a large reprint collection going back to 1914. The Library of the Benjamin Rose Institute in Cleveland, Ohio, is a repository for the papers and publications of the Margaret .pa

Blenker Research Institute there and also has a complete set of the annual reports of the Institute back to 1909.

The Philadelphia Corporation for Aging (PCA) Library has copies of all contracts awarded by PCA (for anyone to consult in preparing future proposals), as well as the PCA archives, and an extensive collection of materials relating to the National Long Term Care Demonstration, or, as it was more popularly known, the channeling project (Kemper and Brown, 1986). The Library of the Philadelphia Geriatric Center has an extensive collection of the papers of Elaine Brody and the publications of other staff members. The Resource Center of the Institute on Aging at Temple University in Philadelphia has a set of the SCAN microfiche. The Library at the Tennessee Commission on Aging has the minutes and manuscripts of the Commission from its founding date of 1963 to the present plus materials relating to aging in Tennessee from the 1950s. The J. W. Crane Memorial Library at Deer Lodge Centre in Winnipeg, Canada has the Microfiche Collection in Gerontology and Geriatrics published in 1986 by Microforms International of Pergamon Press.

Serials Currently Received

The survey asked whether libraries or collections had current holdings of 18 selected gerontology, geriatrics, or long-term care serials titles. At the present time there are over 100 serials titles devoted specifically to gerontology, geriatrics, and long-term care (Hesslein, 1986) and the 18 titles were chosen as representative of the wide range of these specific aspects. The responses of the separate gerontology collections at the academic institutions often did not make it clear whether a title was available at the larger university library or the smaller gerontology collection. In these cases, all mentioned titles were counted as received. Appendix C is a coded list of which of the 73 libraries/collections responding to this survey have current holdings of each of the 18 titles.

Two of the most basic journals in the field are the Gerontologist and the Journals of Gerontology which were currently received by 79 percent and 72 percent respectively. These were the highest totals reported in the survey for any of the 18 titles. There are a lot of newsletters in gerontology and one of the most essential is the Older Americans Report, a weekly reporting of Congressional and AoA actions in aging. Fifty-three percent of the respondents receive it. The Journal of the American Geriatrics Society and Clinics in Geriatric Medicine are the two major clinical journal titles in geriatrics and they are currently held by 36 percent and 19 percent respectively. Provider is one of the major journals for long-term care administrators and 19 percent of the libraries/collections receive it. Neurobiology of Aging and Mechanisms of Ageing and Development are two of the most expensive and specialized journals in the field and 7 percent and 4 percent respectively reported that they currently receive these titles. Ten percent of the respondents did not receive any of the 18 titles on the list.

Owens (1978) also included a list of 18 gerontology serial titles in her survey but only five of her titles are on the list of the present survey. Once again the Gerontologist and the Journal of Gerontology (in 1988 the title was changed to Journals of Gerontology) were the most commonly held titles at 83 percent and 80 percent respectively. The Journal of the American Geriatrics Society was received by 40 percent of Owens' respondents.

Subject Strengths of Collections

The study of aging draws from many different disciplines and their materials. Table 8 shows the subject strengths of

Table 8

Collection Subject Strengths[1] (n = 73)

1.	Caregiving, social services, family issues, etc.	45(62%)
2.	Health care, health promotion, etc.	42(58%)
3.	Long term care	41(56%)
4.	Demographic, census, statistical data, etc.	35(48%)
5.	Medicare/Medicaid, insurance, social security, legal, financial, etc.	35(48%)
6.	Medicine, nursing, rehabilitation, etc.	33(45%)
7.	Administration, including nursing homes, retirement facilities, etc.	31(43%)
8.	Housing, living arrangements, environment and product design, etc.	30(41%)
9.	Policy issues	30(41%)
10.	Government publications	26(36%)
11.	Aging network reports, documents, etc.	25(34%)
12.	Psychology, mental health, counseling, etc.	22(30%)
13.	Dying, death, bereavement	17(23%)
14.	Retirement	16(22%)
15.	Research and statistical methods, etc.	14(19%)
16.	Anthropology, ethnicity, cross-cultural studies, etc.	11(15%)
17.	Physiology, aging process, molecular biology, etc.	10(14%)
18.	Education, program development, planning, etc.	8(11%)
19.	Employment	8(11%)
20.	Consumer materials, including easy-to-read, large-print, etc.	4(6%)
21.	International materials	4(6%)

[1]More than 1 answer is possible.

the libraries/collections surveyed and reflects the wide range of questions these collections are used to answer. Appendix D is a list of subject strengths. Very few of the collections cover all, or even most, of these subject strengths, but it is not uncommon for the librarians of these collections to get questions ranging over all these topics and to have to use all known resources to come up with answers for their clientele.

Demographic and statistical data and the economic and legal issues of long-term care are as important as material on the medical and nursing aspects of caring for aging individuals. Policy and government materials are provided more often than books on mental health and bereavement. Material on research and statistical methods are in demand because many of the clientele using these collections are engaged in research. Cross-cultural material and information about aging in countries other than the United States are rising in demand.

Owens (1978) tabulated 15 different subject strengths for the collections she surveyed. Like the present study, she found that material on health issues was the most frequently provided. Unlike the present study, she found that demographic, economic, and political science materials in aging were only provided by 9 percent of her respondents. This may be because there was very little available in these areas 11 years ago. Owens found that material on aging services, agencies, and programs was provided 31 percent of the time. In the other subject strength categories, the findings of the two surveys are quite similar.

Cataloging and Classification

Eighty-five percent of the collections surveyed catalog their books, 25 percent catalog their journals, and 23 percent catalog other materials such as vertical file contents and audiovisual cassettes, films, etc. Eight percent don't catalog anything.

Thirty-four percent use the Library of Congress classification system, 18 percent use the National Library of Medicine system, 12 percent use Dewey, and the highest percentage, 37 percent, use some other system such as alphabetical by author, or by broad subject categories, or by the headings in the various editions of the Thesaurus of Aging Terminology.

When asked which subject authority list(s) was used, most indicated they used more than one. Thirty-eight percent used Library of Congress subject headings, 26 percent used the Thesaurus of Aging Terminology, and 25 percent used the National Library of Medicine Medical Subject Headings (MeSH). Thirty-eight percent used other subject heading lists such as the National Council on the Aging thesaurus, the Subject Guide to IAC (Information Access Company) Databases, the keyword list to the National Aging Resource Center on Elder Abuse database, the Thesaurus of Psychological Index Terms, or the Thesaurus of ERIC Descriptors. Three percent either used Sears or no subject authority list.

Owens (1978) found that 70 percent of her gerontology/learning resource center collections were cataloged and 91 percent of her special/private collections were not. Fifty percent were cataloged using the Library of Congress classification system and the remainder used either Dewey or their own system.

Services

Responses to this survey gave the impression that many libraries and collections do not regularly record the quantities of the different types of services they provide. In addition, the attempt to obtain both a monthly and an annual total figure for a number of measures of service was misunderstood by many respondents.

Summarizing and drawing conclusions about various types of library services from statistics provided by different libraries/collections is always subject to questions of interpretation. Different libraries/collections often do not define or count things in consistent ways. The responses to this survey and the discussions about services that follows are no different.

Table 9 shows the percentages of each of 16 different types of services offered by the gerontology libraries and collections contributing to the present survey with comparisons to the findings of the AHA and Rafferty surveys. The AHA survey (1991, p. 10) used a list of 27 different services. The 16 different services used for the present survey were taken from the longer AHA list, but omitted those that would be unique to a hospital library setting. Rafferty (1983, pp. 12-13, 34-35) asked her libraries which of 16 services appropriate for networking each provided. Only four of her 16 services were common to the 16 services used for the present survey. The findings of the present survey hold no real surprises.

Reference

Reference is the most frequently provided service, although only 88 percent of the present gerontology libraries and collections said they provided it. This figure is open to interpretation because it is not clear that the large libraries and the small collections are defining "reference" the same way. Comments attached to the responses of the small collections lead to the possible conclusion that reference here means any act of using, referring to, or browsing the collection by any user. The large libraries, on the other hand, use reference in the more traditional, restricted sense to mean an encounter when a user asks a specific question either for some informa-

Table 9
Services Provided[1,2] (n = 68)

Type		AHA survey (ranking)	Rafferty survey (ranking)
1. Reference	60(88%)	98%(1)	
2. Circulation	46(63%)	92%(4)	
3. SDI	39(57%)	67%(6)	44%(7)
4. Database searching--library staff	36(53%)	83%(5)	50%(5)
5. Interlibrary loan borrowing	33(49%)	97%(2)	78%(1)
6. Bibliography preparation	30(44%)	57%(9)	
7. AV distribution	28(41%)	59%(8)	
8. Interlibrary loan lending	26(38%)	92%(3)	
9. Learning or resource center functions	24(35%)	19%(16)	
10. User education, bibliographic instruction, etc.	24(35%)	50%(10)	
11. Indexing, abstracting	15(22%)	16%(19)	31%(11)
12. Centralized purchasing	11(16%)	60%(7)	
13. Archives management, preservation, etc.	8(12%)	14%(23)	
14. Database searching--end users	6(9%)	31%(13)	
15. Microcomputer center	5(7%)	15%(21)	
16. End user training	4(6%)	27%(15)	
17. Other	3(4%)	6%(28)	

[1]More than 1 answer is possible.
[2]Five respondents (7%) did not answer the question.

tion (What are all the books and articles James E. Birren has written?) or about the collection (Where can I find the names of the nursing homes in my area?) and receives an expert answer from another individual.

Table 10 gives detailed information about reference services across all 73 libraries/collections participating in the present survey. They were asked for the total number of questions answered in the one month period of March 1990. Almost half, 48 percent, either didn't keep statistics, provide reference, understand the question, or answer the question. Of the remaining 52 percent, almost half, 23 percent, answered 15 or fewer questions during the survey month. Twelve percent of the total number of respondents answered more than 50 questions in that month. The AHA (1991, p. 9) findings are not too dissimilar although their totals are for a one year period. Most said they answered 200 reference questions in one year. The median was 735. Thirty percent of their respondents didn't answer the question.

The bottom half of Table 10 shows that questions on the demographics and statistics of aging are answered more frequently by gerontology libraries/collections than questions about the behavioral or clinical aspects of aging. The second most frequent type of reference service provided is to locate materials for users, both within and outside the home collection. The high numbers here would seem to indicate a real need for gerontology librarians to share information about their holdings and resources and to come together in periodic collective attempts to keep up with and understand the wide variety of statistics available on aging.

Table 11 gives a further breakdown of which types of libraries/collections are providing the most reference service. As noted in a previous comparison, the number of academic gerontology collections not providing reference service is surprisingly high. The most reference questions are being answered by NRCs and libraries in medical facilities, although

Table 10
Reference

NUMBER OF QUESTIONS ANSWERED IN MARCH 1990[1] (n = 73)	
1-15	17(23%)
16-50	12(16%)
More than 50	9(12%)
None (reference is provided)	1(1%)
Doesn't keep statistics	5(7%)
Doesn't provide reference	12(16%)
Misunderstood question time frame	4(6%)
No answer	13(18%)
MOST FREQUENT TYPES OF QUESTIONS ANSWERED[2,3] (n = 41)	
1. Demographic, statistics	18(44%)
2. Collection holdings, locating materials not held, etc.	16(39%)
3. Psychological, social, ethical issues, etc.	11(27%)
4. Medical, nursing, health care, etc.	10(24%)
5. Consumer issues, local services, reimbursement, legal, etc.	10(24%)
6. AV, curricular, training, program planning materials, etc.	9(22%)
7. Long-term care system, policy and legislative issues, etc.	8(20%)
8. Citation verification, bibliographic styles, etc.	2(5%)
9. Administering long-term care facilities, etc.	1(2%)

[1]Percentages may not equal 100 due to rounding.
[2]More than 1 answer is possible.
[3]Thirty-two respondents (44%) did not answer this question.

Table 11

Number of Reference Questions Answered in March 1990 by Type of Collection[1,2,3,4] (n = 39)

Type (number of cases)	0 (% of questions)	1-15 (% of questions)	16-50 (% of questions)	51+ (% of questions)	Reference not provided (% of type)
Academic (19)	0	5(13%)	3(8%)	1(3%)	5(26%)
Medical (14)	0	1(3%)	0	2(5%)	2(14%)
SUAs/AAAs (13)	0	2(5%)	4(11%)	1(3%)	2(15%)
Associations (9)	1(3%)	3(8%)	1(3%)	2(5%)	1(11%)
GECs (8)	0	5(13%)	1(3%)	0	2(25%)
Research (4)	0	0	2(5%)	0	0
Government (3)	0	1(3%)	0	1(3%)	0
NRCs (3)	0	0	1(3%)	2(5%)	0

[1]Five respondents (7%) don't keep statistics.
[2]Four respondents (6%) misunderstood the question time frame.
[3]Thirteen respondents (18%) didn't answer the question.
[4]Percentages may not equal 100 due to rounding.

none of the numbers in the "more than 50" a month category are high.

Circulation

Circulation of materials is the second most frequently offered service by gerontology libraries and collections, although only 63 percent of them provide it compared to 92 percent of the AHA libraries. The top half of Table 12 gives a more detailed analysis of the circulation services of the gerontology libraries during the one month survey period of March 1990. As with the reference tabulations, a large number, 54 percent, either didn't keep statistics, circulate materials, understand or answer the question. A higher number circulate more materials: 21 percent circulated more than 25 items during the survey month compared with 14 percent who circulated 10 or fewer items during that month.

Owens (1978) found that 73 percent of her libraries circulated materials and that most of them placed restrictions on loans to individuals outside the parent organization. The AHA (1991, p. 9) findings reported a median of 1,141 items circulated for their one year period.

Table 13 gives a further breakdown of the circulation figures for the specific types of gerontology libraries/collections. Those most likely not to circulate materials are NRCs, GECs, association libraries, SUAs/AAAs, and collections in academic gerontology centers. Libraries in medical facilities were among the most likely to circulate their materials and they also reported the highest numbers of circulated materials for the survey month.

Table 12
Circulation and Interlibrary Loans (n = 73)

CIRCULATION IN MARCH 1990[1]	
1-10	10(14%)
11-25	9(12%)
More than 25	15(21%)
Doesn't keep statistics	6(8%)
Doesn't circulate materials	21(29%)
Misunderstood question time frame	2(3%)
No answer	10(14%)

INTERLIBRARY LOANS IN MARCH 1990	Borrowed[1] (% of total sample)	Loaned (% of total sample)
1-5	11(15%)	4(6%)
6-30	10(14%)	8(11%)
More than 30	6(8%)	4(6%)
None (interlibrary loan is provided)	4(6%)	9(12%)
Doesn't provide interlibrary loan	33(45%)	41(56%)
Misunderstood question time frame	2(3%)	1(1%)
No answer	7(10%)	6(8%)

[1] Percentages may not equal 100 due to rounding.

Table 13
Circulation in March 1990 by Type of Collection[1,2,3,4] (n = 34)

Type (number of cases)	1-10 (% with circulation)	11-25 (% with circulation)	26+ (% with circulation)	Circulation not provided (% of type)
Academic (19)	4(12%)	2(6%)	3(9%)	4(21%)
Medical (14)	1(3%)	1(3%)	5(15%)	2(14%)
SUAs/AAAs (13)	3(9%)	2(6%)	2(6%)	3(23%)
Associations (9)	1(3%)	0	2(6%)	5(56%)
GECs (8)	1(3%)	1(3%)	1(3%)	5(63%)
Research (4)	0	2(6%)	0	0
Government (3)	0	1(3%)	1(3%)	0
NRCs (3)	0	0	1(3%)	2(67%)

[1]Six respondents (8%) don't keep statistics.
[2]Two respondents (3%) misunderstood the question time frame.
[3]Ten respondents (14%) didn't answer the question.
[4]Percentages may not equal 100 due to rounding.

Interlibrary Loans

For the gerontology libraries responding to the present survey interlibrary loan (ILL) lending is offered 11 percent less frequently than ILL borrowing. This seems to reflect the fact that many of the collections are small with neither a large enough collection or staff to service incoming ILL requests for photocopies or loans of material from their collection. In addition, the small collections are not as likely to have contributed their holdings to any union list. ILL borrowing and lending rank second and third respectively in the services provided by AHA (1991) libraries. Rafferty (1983) does not distinguish between the two directions of ILL activity in her figures.

The bottom half of Table 12 gives a detailed analysis of the ILL activity of gerontology libraries/collections during March 1990. Once again, over half of the respondents either didn't provide ILL, or understand or answer the question. In comparing the numbers of items borrowed and loaned, more libraries borrowed 1 to 5 items in the survey month than borrowed more than 30, while the numbers of libraries loaning items peaked at the middle range of 6 to 30 loans a month. In the AHA survey (1991, p. 9), the most frequently reported number of ILLs for their survey year was 10 and the median was 317. The most frequently reported number of items borrowed from other libraries was 5, and the median was 621.

When asked if there were charges for ILL services, 25 percent of the gerontology libraries said no. Three percent said all users were charged, 10 percent said some users were charged, and 63 percent didn't answer the question. Of the AHA (1991, p. 9) respondents charging for ILL service, 5 percent said all users were charged and 28 percent said some users were charged. Sixty-three percent said there were no charges.

Tables 14 and 15 give further breakdowns of the borrowed

Table 14

Number of Borrowed Interlibrary Loans (ILL) in March 1990 by Type of Collection[1,2,3] (n = 31)

Type (number of cases)	0 (% of loans)	1-5 (% of loans)	6-30 (% of loans)	31+ (% of loans)	ILLs not borrowed (% of type)
Academic (19)	1(3%)	3(10%)	3(10%)	0	9(47%)
Medical (14)	1(3%)	3(10%)	3(10%)	3(10%)	2(14%)
SUAs/AAAs (13)	1(3%)	3(10%)	1(3%)	1(3%)	6(46%)
Associations (9)	1(3%)	1(3%)	0	1(3%)	6(67%)
GECs (8)	0	1(3%)	1(3%)	0	6(75%)
Research (4)	0	0	0	1(3%)	2(50%)
Government (3)	0	0	1(3%)	0	0
NRCs (3)	0	0	1(3%)	0	2(67%)

[1]Two respondents (3%) misunderstood the question time frame.
[2]Seven respondents (10%) didn't answer the question.
[3]Percentages may not equal 100 due to rounding.

Table 15

Number of Loaned Interlibrary Loans (ILL) in March 1990 by Type of Collection[1,2,3] (n = 25)

Type (number of cases)	0 (% of loans)	1-5 (% of loans)	6-30 (% of loans)	31+ (% of loans)	ILLs not loaned (% of type)
Academic (19)	5(20%)	1(4%)	2(8%)	0	9(47%)
Medical (14)	1(4%)	2(8%)	3(12%)	3(12%)	3(21%)
SUAs/AAAs (13)	1(4%)	0	1(4%)	0	10(77%)
Associations (9)	1(4%)	1(4%)	1(4%)	0	6(67%)
GECs (8)	0	0	1(4%)	0	7(88%)
Research (4)	0	0	0	1(4%)	2(50%)
Government (3)	1(4%)	0	0	0	1(33%)
NRCs (3)	0	0	0	0	3(100%)

[1]One respondent (1%) misunderstood the question time frame.
[2]Six respondents (8%) didn't answer the question.
[3]Percentages may not equal 100 due to rounding.

and loaned ILL figures for the specific types of gerontology libraries/collections for March 1990. Libraries in medical facilities are the most likely to both borrow and loan materials and they do so at the highest numbers. GECs are the least likely to borrow materials on ILL and none of the NRCs loaned materials on ILL.

Database Searching

Fifty-three percent of the gerontology libraries offer mediated database searching by library staff and 9 percent offer end user searching, compared with 83 percent and 31 percent, respectively, of the AHA respondents.

Table 16 shows the number of mediated searches performed by gerontology libraries in March 1990. Thirty-eight percent of the respondents gave usable figures, and these show that most of them completed between 9 and 16 searches during the survey month. For the AHA survey (1991, p. 9), the most frequently reported number of database searches for

Table 16
Database Searching (n = 73)

STAFF DATABASE SEARCHES IN MARCH 1990	
Less than 9	9(12%)
9-16	11(15%)
More than 16	7(10%)
None (staff searching is provided)	1(1%)
Doesn't keep statistics	3(4%)
Doesn't provide database searching	35(48%)
Misunderstood question time frame	2(3%)
No answer	5(7%)

their survey period of one year was 100, with the median at 308.

Four percent of the gerontology libraries, compared to 8 percent of the AHA libraries, charge for all searches. Fifteen percent of the gerontology libraries and 30 percent of the AHA libraries charge some users, and 29 percent and 52 percent, respectively, do not charge for database searches. Fifty-one percent of the gerontology libraries did not answer the question.

Table 17 shows which databases gerontology libraries use and which ones are most frequently used.

The most popular ones, MEDLINE, AgeLine, and PsycINFO or PsycLIT, reflect the traditional interests of medical staff, gerontologists, and students. The use of ABI/INFORM, NEXIS, and DUNS reflect the growing importance of information about the business, economic, and regulatory aspects of long-term care and long-term care administration.

BRS is the most frequently used vendor by gerontology librarians (36 percent), followed by DIALOG (22 percent), the National Library of Medicine (19 percent), CompuServe (7 percent), Mead Data Central (3 percent), H. W. Wilson Co. (3 percent), and other (7 percent).

The most frequent kinds of topics searched by gerontology libraries were medical, pharmaceutical, allied health, nutrition, exercise, etc. (19 percent); psychological, sociological, caregiving, assessment, etc. (16 percent); economic, policy issues, legal and regulatory issues, etc. (12 percent); business, administration, specific company information, etc. (4 percent); legislative histories (3 percent); and other (4 percent). Seven percent didn't see any one particular type predominating and 59 percent didn't answer the question.

None of the libraries surveyed provide access to the several tape data archives in aging: the National Archive of Computerized Data on Aging maintained by the Inter-University Consortium for Political and Social Research in Ann Arbor,

Table 17
Databases Used[1,2] (n = 33)

Database	Used (% doing searches)	Frequently used (% using database)
MEDLINE	26(79%)	21(81%)
AgeLine	24(72%)	14(58%)
PsycINFO or PsycLIT	23(70%)	8(35%)
Sociological Abstracts	19(58%)	4(21%)
Health Planning and Administration	17(52%)	4(24%)
ABI/INFORM	6(18%)	2(33%)
CINAHL	5(15%)	0
NEXIS	4(12%)	3(75%)
ERIC	3(9%)	0
DUNS	2(6%)	2(100%)
Dissertation Abstracts	2(6%)	0
Social Science Citation Abstracts	1(3%)	1(100%)
Chemical Abstracts	1(3%)	1(100%)
Other	6(18%)	0

[1]More than 1 answer is possible.
[2]Forty respondents (55%) do not do searches or did not answer the question.

Michigan; the National Database on Aging maintained by several different aging organizations including the National Association of State Units on Aging and the National Association of Area Agencies on Aging; or the Data Archive for Aging and Adult Development maintained by the Center for the Study of Aging and Human Development at Duke University.

Challenges to Providing Services

Respondents were asked to describe their greatest challenges in providing services to their clientele. The largest challenge by far (32 percent) is in finding the time and staff to do everything. Very often these are one-person libraries and often the "librarian" has additional nonlibrary responsibilities. The second biggest challenge (16 percent) is in keeping up with the diverse literature of gerontology and locating fugitive reports, conference proceedings, government publications, etc. Lack of funding or support by the parent organization was given as a challenge by 12 percent of the respondents. The other challenges were: responding to the urgency of requests (11 percent); obtaining and keeping up with library automation technology, search techniques, etc. (8 percent); processing materials for the collection (8 percent); user orientation and education, and publicizing what the library can offer users (8 percent); keeping up professionally, both as a librarian and a gerontologist (4 percent); managing a library in more than one location, library security, etc. (3 percent); and getting users to return borrowed materials (3 percent). Some of the "other" answers (8 percent) were lack of space and seating for the library/collection, having the library/collection area also serve as a meeting room, and not having better library tools and databases specifically for gerontology and geriatrics.

Public Relations

Thirty-three percent of the gerontology libraries/collections said they used public relations or other marketing techniques to publicize their library, 36 percent specifically said they did not, and 32 percent didn't answer the question. Most of those not publicizing their library/collection said they did not have the staff and/or time to respond to the additional requests for services they were sure would be made if they did engage in PR.

When asked if they had a regular library publication, or a regular library column in another publication, 37 percent said yes, 26 percent said no, and 37 percent didn't answer the question.

Automation

Only about half of all the gerontology libraries/collections have any kind of automated operations. Although it is not clear from the survey responses, a lot of this capability appears to be through the shared use of another system, often either a larger university library system or a microcomputer in another office. Few of the libraries seem to have their own integrated library system.

Appendix E lists hardware and software used. Table 18 shows word processing and other administrative tasks are the most frequently automated and that none of the respondents plan to expand their capabilities in this area. Forty-eight percent of those with automated functions said they offer database searching and 10 percent hope to expand in this area. Several indicated they were hoping to install a LAN system to offer simultaneous searching over a wider geographic area.

Although the numbers are relatively small, the range of typically automated library functions is well represented

Table 18
Automation[1]

Activity	Have[2] (% of responses)	Expect to obtain[3] (% of responses)
Word processing; other administrative tasks	30(49%)	0
Database searching	29(48%)	4(10%)
Cataloging	24(39%)	3(7%)
Serials management	12(20%)	2(5%)
Acquisitions	10(16%)	3(7%)
Interlibrary loan	9(15%)	0
Online catalog	9(15%)	3(7%)
Circulation	7(11%)	3(7%)
Other	3(5%)	4(10%)
No automation	23(38%)	--

[1]More than 1 answer is possible.
[2]Twelve respondents (16%) didn't answer the automation activity question.
[3]Thirty-one respondents (43%) didn't answer the future purchase question.

among the gerontology libraries. With the exception of one area, they are not too different from AHA findings (1991, p. 6). The exception is in the use of automation to process interlibrary loan requests. It is the most frequent use of automation in the AHA libraries and is sixth out of the eight uses in gerontology and geriatrics libraries on Table 18. This is not too difficult to interpret. Many gerontology libraries do not participate in interlibrary loan as described earlier. Of those that do, many do not participate in the OCLC system for online routing of ILL requests. And most are not members of the regional medical library network of the National Library of Medicine and do not, therefore, have access to their DOCLINE system for automatic online routing of ILL requests.

Users

Respondents were given a list of ten different types of library users and were asked to rank these from the type making the most use of the library to the type(s) who didn't use the library at all. The three rankings indicating the most use were grouped together into a "highest use" category, the middle four rankings were grouped together into a "medium use" category, the bottom four into a "lowest use" category, and the nonusers into a "doesn't use" category. Data about the types of users and the amount of use of each is given in Table 19.

For the first five types of users on Table 19, "staff" through "medical personnel," the types with the highest numbers of users were also the ones making the heaviest use of the libraries/collections. For example, "staff" was the largest type of user with 79 percent of the respondents saying they served staff. Of these, 83 percent also said that of all the different types of users of their library/collection, "staff" used it the most. "Administrators" through "public officials," the

Table 19
Users[1,2,3] (n = 73)

Type	Highest use (% of users)	Medium use (% of users)	Lowest use (% of users)	Doesn't use (% of total sample)
Staff	48(83%)	8(14%)	2(3%)	15(21%)
Students	39(74%)	13(25%)	1(2%)	20(27%)
Researchers	28(61%)	13(28%)	5(11%)	27(37%)
Service providers	24(53%)	18(40%)	3(7%)	28(38%)
Medical personnel	22(56%)	11(28%)	6(15%)	34(47%)
Administrators	11(31%)	18(51%)	6(17%)	38(52%)
General public	11(31%)	12(34%)	12(34%)	38(52%)
Public officials	4(19%)	11(52%)	6(29%)	52(71%)
Business persons	1(6%)	8(44%)	9(50%)	55(75%)
Media	0	7(41%)	10(59%)	56(77%)
Faculty	6(86%)	1(14%)	0	66(90%)

[1]More than 1 answer is possible.
[2]Figures represent rankings of amount of use by each type of user, not numbers of users.
[3]Percentages may not equal 100 due to rounding.

next three user types on Table 19, make medium use of the collections, and "business persons" and the "media" make the lowest use.

The last user type on Table 19, "faculty," was not on the list of user types in the survey but is presented on this table since seven respondents wrote it in. It was originally considered as a type but was felt to be too vague in terms of the more specific list that was eventually used and was omitted. The "faculty" figures were not used in any further analysis.

A cross-tabulation was then made in an effort to determine which types of users were the most frequent at which types of libraries/collections. There was a potential of 320 categories in which to put the user data. For example, "staff" had 32 categories: eight different types of library/collections, each with four indications of the amount of use: "highest," "medium," "lowest," and "doesn't use." Each of the ten types of users had 32 possible categories. This spread the data too thin, so the three indications of heaviest, medium, and lowest amount of use were omitted and each specific type of user was looked at only in terms of whether or not they used each specific type of library/collection. This data is still too scattered to be statistically significant, but general trends do occur.

The percentages of heaviest "staff" use was highest at SUAs/AAAs and research libraries. The percentages of heaviest "student" use was highest at NRCs and academic collections. The percentages of heaviest use by "researchers" was highest at government libraries and academic collections. The percentages of heaviest use by "service providers" was highest at association libraries and SUAs/AAAs. The percentages of heaviest "medical personnel" use was highest at GECs and libraries/collections at medical facilities. Medical personnel did not use government libraries at all. The percentages of heaviest use by "administrators" was highest at NRCs and medical libraries. The percentages of heaviest use by the "general public" was highest at SUAs/AAAs and medical libraries. The percentages of heaviest use by "public officials" was highest at NRCs and association libraries. They did not use GECs or, surprisingly, government libraries at all. The percentages of heaviest use by both "business persons" and the "media" was highest at association libraries and NRCs and neither type used government libraries at all.

Networking and Resource Sharing

Gerontology libraries/collections were asked if they were members of any library consortia. Sixteen percent were members of at least one local consortia, 10 percent belonged to at least one regional consortia, 8 percent were members of either a national or state group, 21 percent didn't belong to any consortia, and 52 percent didn't answer the question.

They were then asked if they contributed their monograph or serial holdings to any union lists of holdings. Table 20 shows that very few do.

Respondents were asked if they belonged to any professional organizations. In tabulating these data no distinction was made between personal or institutional memberships.

Of the library organization memberships, 12 percent were members of the Medical Library Association (MLA), 7 percent were members of either the Special Libraries Association (SLA) or a regional library association, 6 percent belonged to a national group other than MLA, SLA, or the American Library Association (ALA), 3 percent belonged to either ALA or a local library group, 38 percent didn't belong to any library association, and 47 percent didn't answer the question.

Of the nonlibrary types of memberships held, 18 percent belonged to at least one professional gerontology association, 5 percent belonged to at least one medical organization, 4 percent belonged to a national psychology or sociology asso-

Table 20
Resource Sharing[1] (n = 73)

Material	Number (% of responses)	None (% of responses)	No answer (% of total sample)
SERIALS		13(50%)	47(64%)
OCLC	3(12%)		
Other national list	4(15%)		
Regional list	2(8%)		
Local list	4(15%)		
Other	0		
MONOGRAPHS		18(62%)	44(60%)
OCLC	8(28%)		
Other national list	1(3%)		
Regional list	1(3%)		
Local list	0		
Other	1(3%)		

[1]Percentages may not equal 100 due to rounding.

ciation, none belonged to any professional community association, and 4 percent belonged to some other professional organization.

All of these membership figures are low compared with the figures reported by the AHA libraries (1991, p. 11). Rafferty (1983, p. 13) reported that 16 percent of her 100 gerontology/geriatrics libraries participated in a formal network like the Veterans Administration institutions network, and that 34 percent participated in informal networks such as those used for interlibrary loans.

GERONTOLOGY/GERIATRICS LIBRARY GROUP

The 73 libraries/collections responding to the present survey were asked if there should be an association of gerontology/geriatrics libraries and librarians. Thirty-four percent said yes, 14 percent weren't sure, 1 percent said no, and 51 percent didn't answer the question. Thirty-two percent (23 respondents) said they would be willing to work to form such an association. Those interested come mostly from the northeastern section of the United States (Connecticut, District of Columbia, Maryland, Massachusetts, New York, and Pennsylvania), three were from the South (Florida, Kentucky, and North Carolina), one was from Ohio, five were from the West (Arizona, California and Oregon), and there were four from Canada. Thirty-six percent of the respondents didn't answer the question about a library group.

To ascertain the feasibility of one possible way to network, the survey asked respondents if they used E-mail and found that 4 percent had at least some acquaintance or experience with it.

The main focus of Rafferty's study published in 1983 was whether there was an interest in and support for a joint formal network including both gerontology and geriatrics libraries.

She found that 92 percent of her 100 respondents favored such a network. Eighty-two percent felt their parent organization would support it, and 86 percent said they would be willing to pay a membership fee.

Fifty percent of her respondents preferred that a planning meeting for such an organization be held in conjunction with the annual meeting of the Gerontological Society of America, 18 percent preferred a meeting in conjunction with SLA's annual conference, 9 percent preferred a meeting at MLA's annual meeting, 6 percent preferred meeting in conjunction with the annual meeting of the Western Gerontological Society (now the American Society on Aging), and 18 percent preferred calling a special unaffiliated meeting for the sole purpose of organizing such a network.

Some respondents in the present survey offered their suggestions about with which parent organization a gerontology/geriatrics libraries group should affiliate. These were similar to Rafferty's findings and were also similar in that no clear consensus seemed apparent. There does, however, seem to be some agreement that there should not be a separate organization of gerontology/geriatrics libraries. Perhaps this issue of affiliation is the biggest factor to overcome in bringing together the 23 respondents who indicated their willingness to help start an official group.

Rafferty's findings for her question on the preferred organizational structure for a network are difficult to interpret as reported. Fifty-five percent preferred a governing committee, 52 percent thought there should be a designated national headquarters, 9 percent thought there should be a network chair, and 7 percent thought the way to begin the network was with the appointment or selection of an ad-hoc committee to study existing small networks and submit a plan to prospective participants.

When asked to rank 15 library activities by importance for a joint network, 95 percent of Rafferty's respondents thought bibliographic projects were the most important, followed by, in decreasing order of importance, interlibrary loan, a union catalog, clearinghouse-type activities, reference, and cataloging.

NEEDED REFERENCE SOURCES/INFORMATION PRODUCTS IN AGING

To suggest possible projects for a gerontology/geriatrics libraries group, respondents were asked what reference sources or information products in gerontology and geriatrics needed to be produced or published. The response to this question was somewhat lighter than expected and may be partially explained by several respondents who said they were not librarians and didn't feel qualified to answer the question.

Eleven percent said they would like better access to gerontology materials and suggested a regularly published gerontology alerting/SDI (selective dissemination of information) or a gerontology current contents-type product. They also called for better indexes and abstracts. Eight percent wanted a more comprehensive database and thesaurus specifically for the field that included citations and search terms for geriatrics as well as for gerontology. Seven percent want better reference materials in aging and one specifically mentioned a need for an ongoing guide to government publications on aging. Seven percent also mentioned other more nonlibrary-type needs such as a more comprehensive audiovisual listing than is currently available through the National Library of Medicine's AVLINE, and a guide to program development specifically in gerontology.

Individual respondents suggested that the newsletters on marketing to older adults be indexed in the business or newsletter databases and that a database on the legal aspects of gerontology, case law in particular, is needed. Several suggestions for directories were made: a comprehensive directory of organizations and resource persons arranged by the individual specific disciplines of gerontology such as Alzheimer's disease, housing, public policy, retirement etc., and a comprehensive U. S. directory of geriatric services. More demographic sourcebooks in gerontology were suggested as well as more interdisciplinary gerontological/geriatric statistical compilations. A reference manual on nursing home procedures was also suggested.

Four percent said more management materials specifically for gerontology/geriatrics libraries are needed and two suggestions were for a basic core collection list for geriatrics and gerontology libraries similar to the Brandon-Hill lists (1991) for medical libraries (after this survey was made, such a volume was published [Brazil, 1990]), and a better overview or quick reference guide to the more commonly used Library of Congress classification numbers in aging now scattered throughout several different Library of Congress classification schedules. Three percent said better bibliographic control and dissemination of information to gerontology libraries about newly issued aging materials in all its relevant disciplines is needed. Surprisingly, only 1 percent mentioned the need to know the holdings of other gerontology/geriatrics libraries through union lists, etc. One respondent suggested that Serials on Aging (Hesslein, 1986) be updated. Sixty-four percent didn't answer the question about needed projects and products.

LIBRARIES OFFERING SUBSTANTIAL SERVICES

Four measures of the survey were chosen as indicators of substantial library service. The 23 collections with at least one full-time professional librarian were analyzed to see which ones were also answering the most reference questions and borrowing or lending the highest amounts of interlibrary loans. A high number for lending materials to other libraries on interlibrary loan would seem to indicate a large library with enough staff to respond to a wider group of users than just their primary clientele. As noted at the beginning of the section on services, some of the figures given by respondents for these measures are subject to questions of interpretation.

Three of the 23 libraries/collections answered more than 50 reference questions and either requested or supplied 30 or more ILL requests in the one-month period of the survey. They are the AARP Research Information Center in Washington, D.C., with nine full-time and one part-time librarians, over 20,000 monograph titles, and over 350 current serial titles; the Philadelphia Geriatric Center Library with one full-time librarian, over 10,000 monograph titles, and over 200 current serial titles; and the J. W. Crane Memorial Library at Deer Lodge Centre in Winnipeg, Canada, with one full-time librarian, over 4,000 monograph titles, and over 185 current serial titles.

Three other libraries answered 50 or more questions but had a somewhat smaller number of ILLs. They are the National Council on the Aging Library in Washington, D.C., with one full-time and three part-time librarians, over 14,000 monograph titles, and almost 300 current serial titles; the City of Chicago Department on Aging and Disability Library with one full-time librarian, almost 4,000 monograph titles, and over 100 current serial titles; and the Ohio State Department of Aging Resource Center in Columbus with one full-time librarian, 2,000 monograph titles, and almost 90 current serial titles.

Two other libraries had 30 or more ILL requests but a somewhat smaller number of reference questions. They are the Gerontology Research Center Library of the National Institute on Aging in Baltimore with one full-time librarian, over 8,000 monograph titles, and over 400 current serial titles; and the Minnesota Department of Human Services Library in St. Paul with one full-time librarian, 5,000 monograph titles, and over 150 current serial titles.

Keeping within the category of having at least one full-time professional librarian and turning to the middle range of numbers of reference questions and ILL requests for the survey month, two libraries/collections provided both reference and ILLs in these ranges. The first is the collection at the University of California, San Francisco, Institute for Health and Aging with one full-time librarian, over 1,000 monograph titles, and 80 current serial titles, but not open to the public. The second collection is at the Gerontology Research Centre at Simon Fraser University in Vancouver, British Columbia, with one full-time librarian, over 5,000 monograph titles, and about 25 current serial titles.

Four libraries/collections provided no reference but processed a middle range of ILLs. They are the libraries at the Andrus Gerontology Center at the University of Southern California in Los Angeles with one full-time librarian, 9,000 monograph titles, and 100 current serial titles; the health sciences library at the Monroe Community Hospital in Rochester, New York, with a special emphasis on geriatrics, gerontology, and long-term care and with one full-time librarian, over 1,000 monograph titles, and almost 200 current serial titles; the Benjamin Rose Institute in Cleveland, Ohio, with one full-time librarian, 3,000 monograph titles, and over 70 current serial titles; and the Baycrest Centre for Geriatric Care in Toronto, Ontario, with one full-time librarian, over 2,000 monograph titles, and over 150 current serial titles.

One library, the Philadelphia Corporation for Aging Library with one full-time librarian, 2,000 monograph titles, and over 40 current serial titles, provided a middle range of reference service, but processed no ILLs.

LIBRARIES ENDURING THROUGH TIME

Another measure of substantial libraries/collections is how well they endure through time. The 1980 Owens Directory of Gerontological Libraries and Information Centers was the first and only directory of this kind. One of the goals of the present survey was to find out which of the libraries identified by Owens were still in existence ten years later and what had happened to those that were not.

Twenty-four of the original 59 identified libraries, or 41 percent, were found to still be functioning. Questionnaires received from 8, or 14 percent, of the libraries/collections indicated they were no longer in existence for the following reasons: 4 said that what had once been a separate gerontology/geriatrics collection had been merged into a larger general collection; 4 more said that the collection was no longer active, maintained, or functioning. Five of the collections, or 8 percent, no longer seem to have a gerontology focus and 22, or 37 percent, of the collections identified in 1980 seem to have simply disappeared.

3

Directory

ARIZONA

AZ-1 PIMA COUNCIL ON AGING. RESOURCE LIBRARY. 2919 East Broadway, Tucson, AZ 85712. Telephone: 602-795-5800

Type: Area Agency on Aging (AAA)

Librarian: Mary C. Guilbert

Staff: 1 professional librarian (part-time), 1 assistant (part-time)

Founded: 1980

Hours: Monday-Friday 1p.m.-5p.m.

Holdings: 100 monographs; 10,000 reports, manuals, government documents; 23 current serial titles; 280 newsletter and newspaper titles; 10 audiocassettes; 20 videocassettes

Subject strengths: Administration; aging network; death and dying; demographic/census/statistics; economic; employment; government documents; health care; living arrangements; long-term care; policy issues; program planning/training; retirement; social services

Services provided: Photocopy machine; reference; alerting/SDI; bibliography preparation; database searching by staff; interlibrary loan (borrowing and lending); circulation (limited); AV distribution

Automation: Microcomputer; Marcon for cataloging, serials management, and online catalog; BRS for database searching; WordPerfect and D-Base III for word processing, etc.

Gerontology/geriatrics libraries organization: Yes; willing to help start

CALIFORNIA

Berkeley

CA-1 ALTA BATES-HERRICK HOSPITAL. VINTAGE HEALTH LIBRARY AND RESOURCE CENTER. 2001 Dwight Way, Berkeley, CA 94705. Telephone: 415-540-4475

Type: Nursing home

Person-in-charge: Maureen Rafferty

Staff: 1 paraprofessional, 2 assistants (part-time), 13 volunteers (part-time)

Founded: 1957

Hours: Tuesday 10a.m.-7p.m., Wednesday-Friday 10a.m.-4p.m.

Holdings: 7 current serial titles; 3 newspaper titles; 30 audiocassettes; 104 videocassettes; 2 pamphlet file drawers

Subject strengths: Consumer materials; death and dying; geriatrics; health care; living arrangements; long-term care; psychology/mental health; retirement; social services

Services provided: Photocopy machine; reference; bibliography preparation; circulation; AV distribution

Automation: Minicomputer; word processing, etc.

Publications: Just for You (newsletter)

Comment: Library is for older health consumers and their families and caregivers.

Emeryville

CA-2 AGE WAVE, INC. LIBRARY. 1900 Powell Street, Suite 800, Emeryville, CA 94608. Telephone: 415-

652-9099. FAX: 415-652-8245
Type: Research
Person-in-charge: Judy Peck
Staff: 1 paraprofessional (part-time), 1 assistant (part-time)
Founded: 1984
Hours: Not open to the public
Holdings: 1,200 monographs; 120 serial and newsletter titles; 80 audiocassettes; 125 videocassettes; 20 pamphlet file drawers
Subject strengths: Demographic/census/statistics; marketing
Services provided: Photocopy machine; reference; database searching by staff
Automation: BRS and DIALOG for database searching
Comment: Private business library.

Los Angeles

CA-3 ASOCIACION NACIONAL PRO PERSONAS MAYORES. LIBRARY. 3325 Wilshire Blvd. Los Angeles, CA 90010-1724. Telephone: 213-487-1922. FAX 213-385-3014
Type: Association
Person-in-charge: Peggy Smith
Staff: 3 paraprofessionals (part-time)
Founded: 1975
Hours: Monday-Friday 9a.m.-5p.m.
Holdings: 2,000 monographs; 30 current serial titles; 4 videocassettes
Subject strengths: Anthropology/ethnicity; demographic/census/statistics; economic; government documents; health care; Hispanic aging and elderly; living arrangements; policy issues

Services provided: Photocopy machine; reference; circulation; AV distribution

Publications: Newsletter

Gerontology/geriatrics libraries organization: Yes; willing to help start

Comment: Also known as the National Association for Hispanic Elderly.

CA-4 UNIVERSITY OF SOUTHERN CALIFORNIA. ANDRUS GERONTOLOGY CENTER. ANDRUS GERONTOLOGY LIBRARY. University Park, Los Angeles, CA 90089-0191. Telephone: 213-746-5990. RLIN code: CSCW

Type: Academic

Librarian: Stella Fu

Staff: 1 professional librarian, 1 paraprofessional, 3 assistants (part-time)

Founded: 1966

Hours: Open 56 hours a week; hours vary according to academic year

Holdings: 9,000 monographs; 105 current serial titles; 300 newsletter titles; 5 audiocassettes; 43 videocassettes; 37,000 microform titles; 15 pamphlet file drawers

Subject strengths: Aging network; death and dying; government documents; living arrangements; policy issues; psychology/mental health; retirement; social services

Special collections: SCAN microfiche collection; material by and about Ethel Percy Andrus

Services provided: Photocopy machine; reference; alerting/SDI; database searching by staff and end users (fee charged for some users); circulation; interlibrary loan (borrowing and lending; fee charged for some users); AV distribution; archives management

Automation: Microcomputer; Geac for acquisitions, serials management, circulation and online catalog; RLIN and OCLC for cataloging and interlibrary loan; BRS, DIALOG, and USCInfo for database searching, ProCite for bibliographic management; Wordstar and WordPerfect for word processing, etc.

Networks: Inter-University Consortium for Political and Social Research (ICPSR); Research Library Group (RLG); Research Library Information Network (RLIN); USC-UCLA-CAL TECH Consortium; USC-CAL STATE LA Network; California Academic Library Listing of Serials (CALLS). Monographs are listed in RLIN since 1985; serial titles are listed in USC Union List of Serials.

Publications: Recent Acquisitions (quarterly acquisitions list)

Gerontology/geriatrics libraries organization: Yes; willing to help start

San Francisco

CA-5 UNIVERSITY OF CALIFORNIA. SAN FRANCISCO. INSTITUTE FOR HEALTH AND AGING. RESOURCE CENTER. 201 Filbert Street, Suite 500, San Francisco, CA 94133. Telephone: 415-362-3620. FAX: 415-362-0258

Type: Academic

Librarian: Ida VSW Red

Staff: 1 professional librarian, 1 assistant

Founded: 1979

Hours: Monday-Friday 8:30a.m.-5p.m. (not open to the public)

Holdings: 1,000 monographs; 80 current serial titles; 10 audiocassettes; 5 videocassettes; 30 microform titles; 75 pamphlet file drawers

Subject strengths: Aging network; demographic/census/statistics; economic; education/training; government documents; health care; health services; living arrangements; long-term care; policy issues; research methods; social services

Services provided: Photocopy machine; reference; alerting/SDI; bibliography preparation; indexing and abstracting; database searching by staff; circulation

Automation: Microcomputer, access to mainframe computer; Melvyl (UC Library system) and MEDLARS for database searching

Publications: Information Centering (semi-monthly in-house acquisitions list); Research Briefs

Gerontology/geriatrics libraries organization: Yes; willing to help start

CONNECTICUT

Farmington

CT-1 UNIVERSITY OF CONNECTICUT GERIATRIC EDUCATION CENTER. TRAVELERS CENTER ON AGING. EDUCATION RESOURCE CENTER. Farmington, CT 06032. Telephone: 203-679-3956

Type: Academic

Person-in-charge: Amy Louise Frey

Staff: 1 paraprofessional (part-time), 1 assistant (part-time)

Founded: 1986

Hours: Monday-Friday 8:30a.m.-12:30p.m.

Holdings: No collection on site; uses the resources of the University of Connecticut Health Center, Lyman

Maynard Stowe Library, at Farmington

Services provided: Reference; alerting/SDI; bibliography preparation; indexing/abstracting; database searching by staff and end users

Automation: Microcomputer; BRS and MEDLARS for database searching; ProCite for bibliographic management

Publications: Current Literature in Geriatrics and Gerontology

Gerontology/geriatrics libraries organization: Yes; willing to help start

Newington

CT-2 HARTFORD HOSPITAL. JEFFERSON HOUSE. GERONTOLOGY RESOURCE CENTER. 1 John H. Stewart Drive, Newington, CT 06111. Telephone: 203-667-4453. FAX: 203-525-0398. OCLC code: HOS

Type: Medical/nursing home

Librarian: Virginia H. Corcoran

Staff: 1 professional librarian (part-time), 1 volunteer (part-time)

Founded: 1981

Hours: Staffed 20 hours a week; key available at other times

Holdings: 750 monographs; 52 current serial titles; 11 audiocassettes; 70 videocassettes; 3 pamphlet file drawers

Subject strengths: Administration; employment; geriatrics; health care; living arrangements; long-term care; policy issues; retirement; social services

Services provided: Photocopy machine; reference; alerting/SDI; bibliography preparation; indexing and abstracting; database searching by staff; circulation; interlibrary loan (borrowing and lending); AV distribution

Automation: Minicomputer; Hartford Hospital Health Science Libraries shared network/utility for acquisitions and OCLC access for cataloging and online catalog; REMO (ReadMore) for serials management; Smartcom for access to BRS, DIALOG, MEDLARS, and CompuServe for database searching; DOCLINE for interlibrary loan; WordPerfect for word processing, etc.; Ventura for desktop publishing; ProCite and Sci-Mate for bibliographic and information management

Networks: Consortium for Education in Long Term Care Facilities (local); Connecticut Association of Health Science Libraries (CAHSL); Connecticut Association of Non-Profit Facilities for Aged - In Service Education.

Monographs are listed in OCLC; serial titles are listed in SERHOLD (National Library of Medicine).

Publications: GeriSource (newsletter issued 3 times a year); brochures for special programs; information sheets on special aging topics

Gerontology/geriatrics libraries organization: Yes; willing to help start

DELAWARE

DE-1 DELAWARE. DIVISION OF AGING. LIBRARY. 1901 North DuPont Highway, New Castle, DE 19720. Telephone: 302-421-6791. FAX: 302-421-6086

Type: State Unit on Aging and Area Agency on Aging (SUA/AAA)

Person-in-charge: Gloria James
Staff: 1 paraprofessional
Founded: 1973
Hours: Monday-Friday 8a.m.-4:30p.m.
Holdings: 15 current serial titles; 4 newspaper titles; 8 audiocassettes; 43 videocassettes; 16mm films
Subject strengths: Aging network; economic; government documents; health care; physiology; training
Services provided: Photocopy machine; AV distribution
Publications: Periodic updates of information available in the library

DISTRICT OF COLUMBIA

DC-1 AMERICAN ASSOCIATION OF RETIRED PERSONS. RESEARCH INFORMATION CENTER. 601 E Street NW, Building A, 2nd floor, Washington, DC 20049. Telephone: 202-434-6240. FAX: 202-434-6451. OCLC code: NGR
Type: Association
Librarian: Paula M. Lovas
Staff: 10 professional librarians (1 part-time), 7 assistants
Founded: 1964
Hours: Monday-Friday 9a.m.-5p.m.
Holdings: 20,000 monographs; 350 current serial titles; 6 newspaper titles; 50 microform titles; 1 locally mounted database; 15 pamphlet file drawers
Subject strengths: Aging network; anthropology/ethnicity; demographic/census/statistics; economic; employment; government documents; health care; living arrangements; international; long-term care; policy issues; psychology/mental health; retirement; social services

Special collections: 1971 and 1981 White House Conferences on Aging; hearings and reports of U.S. Senate and House of Representatives Special Committees on Aging

Services provided: Photocopy machine; reference; alerting/SDI; bibliography preparation; indexing and abstracting; database producer; database searching by staff and end users; circulation; interlibrary loan (borrowing and lending); archives management

Automation: Microcomputer; minicomputer; STAR for acquisitions, circulation, and online catalog; OCLC and STAR for cataloging; OCLC for interlibrary loan; AARP shared system for serials management, word processing, etc.; BRS, DIALOG, Westlaw, Mead Data Central, LegiSlate, VU/TEXT, Dow Jones News/Retrieval, and CompuServe for database searching; ProCite for bibliographic management

Networks: CAPCON Library Network.
Monographs are listed in OCLC.

Publications: Daily Press Review (in-house); Weekly Journal Contents Service (in-house); Accessions (monthly); Acronyms in Aging (every 3 years)

DC-2 AMERICAN ASSOCIATION OF RETIRED PERSONS. NATIONAL RESOURCE CENTER ON HEALTH PROMOTION AND AGING. 1909 K Street NW, 5th floor, Washington, DC 20049. Telephone: 202-728-4476

Type: National resource center (NRC)

Person-in-charge: Kathleen Nelson

Staff: 1 paraprofessional, 1 assistant (part-time)

Founded: 1988

Hours: Monday-Friday 10a.m.-5p.m. (by appointment)

Subject strengths: Health care and promotion

Services provided: Reference; bibliography preparation; indexing/abstracting; database searching by staff

Automation: Minicomputer; AARP shared system for cataloging, database searching, word processing, etc.

Publications: Perspectives in Health Promotion and Aging (newsletter); individual health promotion information sheets on specific topics

Comment: Referral service and nonlending resource center for health and aging professionals in the aging network.

DC-3 NATIONAL ALLIANCE OF SENIOR CITIZENS. LIBRARY. 1700 18th Street NW, Suite 401, Washington, DC 20009. Telephone: 202-986-0117.

Type: Association

Person-in-charge: Lawrence Bivins

Staff: 1 paraprofessional (part-time)

Founded: 1974

Hours: Monday-Friday 9a.m.-5:30p.m.

Holdings: 1,200 monographs; 5 current serial titles; 5 videocassettes

Subject strengths: Administration; economic; government documents; health care; policy issues

Services provided: Photocopy machine

DC-4 NATIONAL COUNCIL ON THE AGING, INC. OLLIE A. RANDALL LIBRARY. 409 Third Street SW, 2nd floor, Washington, DC 20024. Telephone: 202-479-6665. FAX: 202-479-0735

Type: Association

Librarian: Janette Hoisington

Staff: 4 professional librarians (3 part-time)

Founded: 1950

Hours: Tuesday-Friday 9a.m.-5p.m.

Holdings: 14,000 monographs; 275 current serial titles; 32 pamphlet file drawers

Subject strengths: Administration; death and dying; economic; employment; geriatrics; health care; living arrangements; long-term care; policy issues; retirement; social gerontology; social services

Special collections: Ollie A. Randall papers

Services provided: Photocopy machine; reference; alerting/SDI; bibliography preparation; indexing and abstracting; circulation; interlibrary loan (borrowing and lending)

Automation: Minicomputer; NCOA shared system for word processing

Networks: Federal Library and Information Network (FEDLINK)

Publications: Abstracts in Social Gerontology (quarterly; published by Sage Publications)

Gerontology/geriatrics libraries organization: Yes; willing to help start

DC-5 NATIONAL COUNCIL OF SENIOR CITIZENS. INFORMATION CENTER. 925 15th Street NW, Washington, DC 20005. Telephone: 202-347-8800. FAX: 202-624-9595

Type: Association

Librarian: Brien Kinkel

Staff: 1 professional librarian, 1 assistant

Founded: 1974

Hours: Monday-Friday 9a.m.-5p.m.

Holdings: 3,000 monographs; 200 current serial titles; 8 newspaper titles; 24 videocassettes; 18 pamphlet file drawers

Subject strengths: Demographic/census/statistics; economic; government documents; living arrangements;

policy issues

Services provided: Photocopy machine; reference; alerting/SDI; database searching by staff

Automation: Microcomputer; DIALOG and Washington Alert for database searching

Publications: Acquisitions List (monthly)

DC-6 SOCIAL SECURITY ADMINISTRATION. DISTRICT OF COLUMBIA BRANCH LIBRARY. 4301 Connecticut Avenue NW, Washington, DC 20008. Telephone: 202-282-7179 or 282-7000. FAX: 202-282-7219

Type: Government

Librarian: Linda DelBene

Staff: 1 professional librarian (part-time), 1 assistant (part-time)

Founded: 1972

Hours: Monday-Friday 8:30a.m.-5:30 p.m.

Holdings: 10,000 monographs; 175 current serial titles; 4 newspaper titles; 55 microform titles; 1 pamphlet file drawer

Subject strengths: Demographic/census/statistics; economic; policy issues; research methods; retirement

Services provided: Photocopy machine; reference; alerting/SDI; database searching by staff; circulation; interlibrary loan (borrowing and lending)

Automation: Microcomputer; Social Security Administration's headquarters library's (in Baltimore) shared network/utility used for acquisitions, cataloging, and online catalog; Mead Data Central's NEXIS used for database searching; RWord used for word processing, etc.

Networks: Monographs and serial titles are listed in OCLC.

Gerontology/geriatrics libraries organization: Yes

FLORIDA

Gainesville

FL-1 UNIVERSITY OF FLORIDA. CENTER FOR GERONTOLOGICAL STUDIES. REFERENCE LIBRARY. 3355 Turlington Hall, Gainesville, FL 32611-2036. Telephone: 904-392-2116. FAX: 904-392-6929

Type: Academic

Person-in-charge: Tanya Woolery

Staff: 2 assistants (part-time)

Founded: 1978

Hours: Monday-Friday 9a.m.-4p.m.

Holdings: 12 current serial titles; 11 newsletter titles; 8 videocassettes; (uses collection at main university library for most items)

Subject strengths: Administration; death and dying; demographic/census/statistics; geriatrics; health care; research methods; retirement

Services provided: Photocopy machine; reference; database searching by staff; circulation; Geron-TEL (national phone service providing information on topics related to aging)

Miami

FL-2 UNIVERSITY OF MIAMI SCHOOL OF MEDICINE. CENTER FOR ADULT DEVELOPMENT AND AGING/MIAMI AREA GERIATRIC EDUCATION CENTER. U.M. POMERANCE LIBRARY AND RESOURCE CENTER. P.O. Box 016960, Miami, FL 33101. Telephone: 305-326-1043. FAX: 305-

545-9435. OCLC code: FQMJ
Type: Medical
Librarian: Carmen B. Rivera
Staff: 1 professional librarian, 1 assistant (part-time)
Founded: 1986
Hours: Monday-Friday 9a.m.-5p.m.
Holdings: 322 monographs; 20 current serial titles; 15 newsletter titles; 1 newspaper title; 35 audiocassettes; 38 videocassettes; 1 CD-ROM title; 2 pamphlet file drawers
Subject strengths: Aging network; anthropology/ethnicity; demographic/census/statistics; geriatric education; geriatrics; health care; physiology; psychology/mental health; research methods; social services
Services provided: Photocopy machine; reference; alerting/SDI; bibliography preparation; indexing and abstracting; database searching by staff and end users (fee charged for some users); circulation; interlibrary loan (borrowing and lending; fee charged for some users); AV distribution
Automation: Microcomputer; CD-ROM drive; OCLC terminal software for cataloging; Innovative Interface's Innopac for circulation and online catalog; BRS Colleague, PaperChase, SilverPlatter, and CompuServe for database searching; ProCite for bibliographic management; WordPerfect, DBase and Lotus for word processing, budgets, etc.
Networks: Southeastern Library Network (SOLINET). Monographs and audiovisual titles are listed in OCLC.
Publications: Training and Educational Resources in Geriatrics (annual)
Gerontology/geriatrics libraries organization: Yes; willing to help start

Pensacola

FL-3 UNIVERSITY OF WEST FLORIDA. CENTER ON AGING. DEPARTMENT OF SOCIAL WORK. 11000 University Parkway, Pensacola, FL 32514. Telephone: 904-474-2381. FAX: 904-474-3130

Type: Academic

Person-in-charge: Carol Rafalski

Staff: 1 paraprofessional (part-time)

Founded: 1982

Hours: Monday-Friday 8a.m.-4:30p.m.

Holdings: 50 monographs; 3 current serial titles

Subject strengths: Death and dying; demographic/census/statistics; economic; geriatrics; government documents

Services provided: Reference; circulation

Tampa

FL-4 UNIVERSITY OF SOUTH FLORIDA. SUNCOAST GERONTOLOGY CENTER. EASTERN STAR LIBRARY ON ALZHEIMER'S DISEASE. 12901 North 30th Sreet, Tampa, FL 33617. Telephone: 813-974-4355. FAX: 813-974-4251

Type: Academic

Librarian: Susan M. Quinn

Staff: 1 professional librarian, 1 paraprofessional

Founded: 1990

Hours: Monday-Friday 8:30a.m.-4:30p.m.

Holdings: 500 monographs; 200 videocassettes; 6 pamphlet file drawers

Subject strengths: Alzheimer's disease; long-term care; psychology/mental health; social services

Services provided: Photocopy machine; reference; alerting/SDI; bibliography preparation; indexing/abstracting; database searching by staff (fee charged for some users); circulation

Automation: Microcomputer; LUIS for online catalog; DIALOG for database searching; Microsoft Word and DBase for word processing, etc.

Networks: Tampa Bay Medical Library Network

Publications: Alzheimer's Resource News (semi-annual)

Comment: Also the National Resource Center on Alzheimer's Disease.

HAWAII

HI-1 PACIFIC ISLANDS GERIATRIC EDUCATION CENTER. REFERENCE LIBRARY. University of Hawaii Kuakini Medical Center, 347 N. Kuakini Street, HPM 9, Honolulu, HI 96817. Telephone: 808-523-8461. FAX: 808-523-8969

Type: Geriatric education center (GEC)

Person-in-charge: Nathan Kwon

Staff: 1 assistant (part-time)

Founded: 1987

Hours: Monday-Friday 9a.m.-5p.m.

Holdings: 40 current serial titles; 45 videocassettes; 6 pamphlet file drawers

Subject strengths: Administration; aging network; anthropology/ethnicity; death and dying; demographic/census/statistics; economic; geriatrics; government documents; health care; living arrangements; international; long-term care; physiology; policy issues; psychology/mental health; research methods; social services

Services provided: Photocopy machine

Automation: Microcomputer

ILLINOIS

Chicago

IL-1 CITY OF CHICAGO. DEPARTMENT ON AGING AND DISABILITY. LIBRARY. 510 North Peshtigo Court, 38, Chicago, IL 60611. Telephone: 312-744-1686

Type: Area Agency on Aging (AAA)

Librarian: Kalina Pomirko

Staff: 1 professional librarian, 1 assistant (part-time)

Founded: 1972

Hours: Monday-Friday 8:30a.m.-4:30p.m.

Holdings: 3750 monographs; 35 current serial titles; 70 newsletter titles; 4 newspaper titles; 100 videocassettes; 125 microform titles; 52 pamphlet, document, agency records, etc. file drawers

Subject strengths: Demographic/census/statistics; economic; government documents; living arrangements; policy issues; social services

Services provided: Reference; alerting/SDI; circulation; interlibrary loan (borrowing only); AV distribution

IL-2 GREAT LAKES GERIATRIC EDUCATION CENTER. RESOURCE CENTER. Chicago College of Osteopathic Medicine, 5200 South Ellis Avenue, Chicago, IL 60615. Telephone: 312-947-3386

Type: Geriatric education center (GEC)

Person-in-charge: J. M. Doherty-Greenberg

Staff: 2 paraprofessionals (part-time)

Founded: 1987

Hours: Monday-Friday 9a.m.-5p.m.

Holdings: 850 monographs; 33 newsletter titles; 36 videocassettes; 8 pamphlet file drawers

Subject strengths: Death and dying; demographic/census/statistics; economic; psychology/mental health; retirement

Services provided: Photocopy machine; reference

KANSAS

KS-1 KANSAS STATE UNIVERSITY. CENTER FOR AGING. GERONTOLOGY LIBRARY. Fairchild Hall, Room 1, Manhattan, KS 66506. Telephone: 913-532-5945. FAX: 913-532-5944

Type: Academic

Person-in-charge: Edith Stunkel

Staff: 1 volunteer (part-time)

Founded: 1975

Hours: Monday-Friday 8a.m.-5p.m.

Holdings: 80 audiocassettes; 28 videocassettes (monographs and archives have been moved to the main university library)

Services provided: AV distribution

KENTUCKY

KY-1 OHIO VALLEY APPALACHIA REGIONAL GERIATRIC EDUCATION CENTER. University of Kentucky, Sanders-Brown Center on Aging, 20 Medical Center Annex 1, Lexington, KY 40536-0079. Telephone: 606-257-5915. FAX: 606-258-2866

Type: Geriatric education center (GEC)
Librarian: Peter Taylor
Staff: 1 professional librarian (part-time), 1 assistant (part-time)
Founded: 1985
Hours: Monday-Friday 8a.m.-4:30p.m.
Holdings: 220 monographs; 2 current serial titles; 30 newsletter titles; 2 audiocassettes; 37 videocassettes; 2 pamphlet file drawers; 8 films; 3 simulation games
Subject strengths: Aging network; geriatric education; geriatrics
Services provided: Photocopy machine; reference; alerting/SDI; bibliography preparation; database searching by staff (fee charged for some users); circulation; AV distribution
Automation: BRS for database searching
Gerontology/geriatrics libraries organization: Yes; willing to help start

MARYLAND

Baltimore

MD-1 NATIONAL INSTITUTE ON AGING. GERONTOLOGY RESEARCH CENTER LIBRARY. 4940 Eastern Avenue, Baltimore, MD 21224. Telephone: 410-558-8124. FAX: 410-558-8103. OCLC code: GRL
Type: Research
Librarian: Joanna Chen Lin
Staff: 1 professional librarian, 1 paraprofessional (part-time), 2 assistants (part-time)
Founded: 1968

Hours: Monday-Friday 8:30a.m.-5p.m.
Holdings: 8,000 monographs; 418 current serial titles; 7 microform titles; 1 CD-ROM title
Subject strengths: Administration; aging network; anthropology/ethnicity; demographic/census/statistics; economic; employment; geriatrics; health care; living arrangements; long-term care; physiology; psychology/mental health; research methods; retirement
Special collections: Monographs of many early gerontological researchers; bibliographies compiled by Nathan W. Shock
Services provided: Photocopy machine; CD-ROM drive; reference; alerting/SDI; database searching by staff and end users; circulation; interlibrary loan (borrowing and lending)
Automation: Microcomputer; mainframe computer; OCLC workstation for cataloging; REMO (Read-More) for serials management; BRS, DIALOG, STN and MEDLINE (CD Plus) for database searching; ProCite for bibliographic management; Word Perfect and DBase for word processing, etc.
Networks: National Library of Medicine Regional Medical Library Network; Maryland Association of Health Science Librarians (MAHSL); Federal Library and Information Network (FEDLINK). Monographs are listed in OCLC; serial titles are listed in SERLINE (National Library of Medicine), Maryland Interlibrary Organization (MILO), and MAHSL.
Publications: GERON, NIA's monthly newsletter, lists new library acquisitions
Gerontology/geriatrics libraries organization: Yes; willing to help start

MD-2 SOCIAL SECURITY ADMINISTRATION. LIBRARY. P.O. Box 17330, Baltimore, MD 21235. Telephone: 301-965-6109. FAX: 301-965-9956. OCLC code: SSL

Type: Government

Librarian: Joyce Donohue

Staff: 5 professional librarians, 4 paraprofessionals

Founded: 1942

Hours: Monday-Friday 8:30a.m.-5p.m.

Holdings: 30,000 monographs; 400 serial titles

Subject strengths: Administration; demographic/census/statistics; economic; policy issues; retirement

Services provided: Photocopy machine; reference; alerting/SDI; bibliography preparation; indexing and abstracting; database searching by staff and end users (fee charged for all searches); circulation; interlibrary loan (borrowing and lending)

Automation: Microcomputer; minicomputer; OCLC used for acquisitions, cataloging, circulation, and interlibrary loan; BRS, DIALOG, WilsonLine, and CompuServe used for database searching

Networks: Titles are listed in OCLC

MASSACHUSETTS

Boston

MA-1 BOSTON UNIVERSITY. GERONTOLOGY CENTER. LOUIS LOWY LIBRARY IN GERONTOLOGY. 67 Bay State Road, Boston, MA 02215. Telephone: 617-353-5045

Type: Academic

Person-in-charge: Elizabeth Markson

Staff: 1 paraprofessional (part-time)
Founded: 1974
Hours: Monday-Friday 9a.m.-5p.m.
Holdings: 6 current serial titles; 4 videocassettes; 21 pamphlet file drawers
Subject strengths: Economic; health care; living arrangements; long-term care; psychology/mental health; retirement; social services
Services provided: Photocopy machine; reference
Automation: WordPerfect for word processing, etc.

MA-2 USDA (U.S. DEPARTMENT OF AGRICULTURE) HUMAN NUTRITION RESEARCH CENTER ON AGING AT TUFTS UNIVERSITY. LIBRARY. 711 Washington Street, Boston, MA 02111. Telephone: 617-556-3173. FAX: 617-556-3344. OCLC code: USQ
Type: Research
Person-in-charge: Kathleen L. Cappellano
Staff: 1 paraprofessional, 1 assistant (part-time)
Founded: 1977
Hours: Monday-Friday 9a.m.-5p.m. (staff may use at other hours)
Holdings: 474 monographs; 48 current serial titles; 13 newsletter titles; 4 audiocassettes; 8 pamphlet file drawers
Subject strengths: Demographic/census/statistics; geriatrics; nutrition; physiology; research methods
Special collections: Reprints from 13 Human Nutrition Research Center laboratories from 1979 to date
Services provided: Photocopy machine; reference; alerting/SDI; bibliography preparation; database searching by staff (fee charged for all users); circulation; AV distribution; archives management
Automation: Microcomputer; Tufts University Library

shared network/utility used for cataloging, online catalog, and interlibrary loan; BRS and MEDLARS for database searching; WordPerfect, Wordstar, and Lotus for word processing, budgets, etc.

Networks: Boston Library Consortium. Monographs are listed in OCLC.

Waltham

MA-3 BRANDEIS UNIVERSITY. HELLER GRADUATE SCHOOL. HEALTH POLICY CENTER. LIBRARY. Waltham, MA 02254-9110. Telephone: 617-736-3920

Type: National resource center (NRC)

Person-in-charge: Sylvia F. Pendleton

Staff: 1 paraprofessional (part-time), 1 assistant (part-time)

Founded: 1980

Hours: Monday-Friday 9a.m.-5p.m.

Holdings: 2,000 monographs; 61 current serial titles; 1 pamphlet file drawer

Subject strengths: Demographic/census/statistics; economic; government documents; health care; long-term care; policy issues; social services

Services provided: Reference; alerting/SDI; indexing and abstracting; database searching by staff; circulation

Automation: Microcomputer; WPS-PC for word processing

Publications: New Documents (weekly, biweekly, and monthly lists)

Gerontology/geriatrics libraries organization: Yes

Comment: Also the National Resource Center on Long-Term Care.

MICHIGAN

Ann Arbor

MI-1 THE CENTER FOR SOCIAL GERONTOLOGY, INC. LIBRARY. 117-N First Street, Suite 204, Ann Arbor, MI 48104. Telephone: 313-665-1126. FAX: 313-665-2071.

Type: Association

Person-in-charge: Susan Herman

Staff: 1 paraprofessional

Founded: 1971

Hours: Monday-Friday 8:30a.m.-5:30p.m.

Holdings: 15 monographs; 3 current serial titles; 2 videocassettes; 15 pamphlet file drawers

Subject strengths: Administration; aging network; economic; health care; legal aspects; living arrangements; long-term care

Services provided: Photocopy machine

Comment: A National Support Center in Law and Aging.

MI-2 HERMAN MILLER RESEARCH CORPORATION. LIBRARY. 3971 South Research Park Drive, Ann Arbor. MI 48108 Telephone: 313-994-0200. FAX: 313-994-3050

Type: Research

Librarian: Dallas Moore

Staff: 1 professional librarian

Founded: 1987

Hours: Monday-Friday 8:30a.m.-5p.m.

Subject strengths: Living arrangements; long-term care; social services

Services provided: Photocopy machine; reference; alerting/SDI; bibliography preparation; indexing and abstracting; database searching by staff; circulation; interlibrary loan (borrowing only); archives management

Automation: Microcomputer; ProCite for cataloging; BRS and DIALOG for database searching; Microsoft Word for word processing, etc.

Comment: Developer of MetaForm, a research and development program to design and identify products leading to greater independence for aging and disabled people. The library is for corporate use only, but is willing to share nonproprietary information.

Detroit

MI-3 DETROIT AREA AGENCY ON AGING. LIBRARY. 1100 Michigan Building, 220 Bagley, Detroit, MI 48226. Telephone: 313-222-5330

Type: Area Agency on Aging (AAA)

Person-in-charge: Mike Simowski

Staff: 1 paraprofessional (part-time)

Founded: 1980

Hours: Monday-Friday 8:30a.m.-5p.m.

Holdings: 250 monographs; 20 current serial titles; 20 newsletter titles; 12 videocassettes

Subject strengths: Administration; consumer materials; government documents; health care; policy issues

Services provided: Photocopy machine; reference; alerting/SDI; circulation; interlibrary loan (borrowing only); AV distribution

Grand Rapids

MI-4 AREA AGENCY ON AGING OF WESTERN MICHIGAN, INC. REFERENCE AND AUDIOVISUAL LIBRARY. Two Fountain Place, Suite 540, Grand Rapids, MI 49341. Telephone: 616-456-5664. FAX: 616-456-5692

Type: Area Agency on Aging (AAA)

Person-in-charge: Sandra L. Davis

Staff: 1 volunteer (part-time)

Founded: 1977

Hours: Monday-Friday 9a.m.-5p.m.

Holdings: 2,250 monographs; 9 current serial titles; 15 audiocassettes; 27 videocassettes

Subject strengths: Aging network; demographic/census/statistics; economic; government documents; living arrangements; long-term care; research methods; social services

Services provided: Photocopy machine; reference; circulation; AV distribution

Southfield

MI-5 REGION 1-B AREA AGENCY ON AGING. LIBRARY. 29508 Southfield Road, Suite 100, Southfield, MI 48076. Telephone: 313-569-0333. FAX: 313-569-7944

Type: Area Agency on Aging (AAA)

Person-in-charge: Colleen Blaesing

Staff: 1 professional librarian (part-time), 1 paraprofessional (part-time)

Founded: 1974
Hours: Monday-Friday 8:30a.m.-4:30p.m.
Holdings: 500 monographs; 20 current serial titles; 40 videocassettes
Subject strengths: Administration; economic; government documents; policy issues; social services
Services provided: Alerting/SDI; circulation

MINNESOTA

MN-1 MINNESOTA. DEPARTMENT OF HUMAN SERVICES. LIBRARY. 444 Lafayette Road, St. Paul, MN 55155-3821. Telephone: 612-297-8708. OCLC code: DHS
Type: Government
Librarian: Colleen Spadaccini
Staff: 1 professional librarian, 1 assistant, 2 volunteers (part-time)
Founded: 1924
Hours: Monday-Friday 8a.m.-4:30p.m.
Holdings: 5000 monographs; 160 current serial titles; 1 newspaper title; 10 audiocassettes; 150 videocassettes; 10 pamphlet file drawers
Subject strengths: Administration; geriatrics; health care; long-term care; psychology/mental health; social services
Services provided: Photocopy machine; reference; alerting/SDI; bibliography preparation; database searching by staff (fee charged for some users); circulation; interlibrary loan (borrowing and lending; fee charged for some users); AV distribution
Automation: Microcomputer; minicomputer; OCLC for cataloging; PALS (Unisys) for online catalog; Minnesota Interlibrary Telecommunication Network

(MINITEX) and DOCLINE (National Library of Medicine) for interlibrary loan; BRS and DIALOG for database searching; PFS Write, Appleworks, and DBase for word processing, etc.

Networks: Headquarters of Minnesota Department of Human Services Library Consortium; Greater Midwest Regional Medical Library Network; Capitol Area Library Consortium, Metronet.

Monographs and serial titles are listed in OCLC.

MISSOURI

MO-1 UNIVERSITY OF MISSOURI-COLUMBIA. SOCIAL AND BEHAVIORAL SCIENCES REFERENCE CENTER. Medical Sciences Building, Columbia, MO 65212. Telephone: 314-882-6184

Type: Academic

Librarian: Beatrice Engley

Staff: 1 professional librarian, 1 paraprofessional (part-time)

Founded: 1975

Hours: Monday-Friday 7:30a.m.-1:30a.m. and other variable hours

Holdings: 2,400 monographs; 40 current serial titles; 20 pamphlet file drawers

Subject strengths: Administration; anthropology/ethnicity; economic; health care; living arrangements; long-term care; policy issues; retirement; social services

Services provided: Reference; alerting/SDI; bibliography preparation; indexing/abstracting; database searching by staff; circulation; interlibrary loan (borrowing and lending)

Automation: BRS and MEDLARS for database searching are accessed at the University of Missouri-Columbia Medical Center's Health Sciences Library.

Comment: The resource materials of the Center for the Study of Aging at the University of Missouri-Columbia are maintained at the Social and Behavioral Sciences Reference Center of the Department of Family and Community Medicine of the University of Missouri-Columbia's School of Medicine.

NEBRASKA

NE-1 UNIVERSITY OF NEBRASKA AT OMAHA. DEPARTMENT OF GERONTOLOGY. PRIVATE DEPARTMENT COLLECTION. Omaha, NE 68182. Telephone: 402-554-2272

Type: Academic

Person-in-charge: James A. Thorson

Founded: 1972

Hours: Monday-Friday 8a.m.-5p.m. (not open to the public)

Holdings: 500 monographs; 6 current serial titles; 12 audiocassettes; 40 videocassettes

Subject strengths: Death and dying; psychology/mental health; social services

Services provided: Photocopy machine; reference; database searching by end users

Automation: Microcomputer

NEW YORK

Albany

NY-1 CENTER FOR THE STUDY OF AGING. LIBRARY. 706 Madison Avenue, Albany, NY 12208. Telephone: 518-465-6927 or 462-1331. FAX: 518-462-1339

Type: Association

Person-in-charge: Sara Harris

Staff: 1 paraprofessional (part-time)

Founded: 1957

Hours: by appointment only

Holdings: 4,000 monographs; 5 current serial titles; 10 audiocassettes; 15 videocassettes; 20 pamphlet file drawers

Subject strengths: Death and dying; geriatrics; living arrangements; physical fitness/wellness; psychology and mental health; social services

Services provided: Photocopy machine; reference; alerting/SDI

Automation: Microcomputer

Buffalo

NY-2 WESTERN NEW YORK GERIATRIC EDUCATION CENTER. RESOURCE CENTER. State University of New York at Buffalo, Beck Hall, 3435 Main Street, Buffalo, NY 14214. Telephone: 716-831-3176. FAX: 716-831-2308

Type: Geriatric education center (GEC)

Person-in-charge: Lisa A. Nolan

Staff: 1 paraprofessional (part-time)

Founded: 1983

Hours: Monday-Friday 9a.m.-5p.m.

Holdings: 25 current serial titles; 10 videocassettes; 5 pamphlet file drawers

Subject strengths: Aging network; demographic/census/statistics; economic; geriatrics; government documents; health care; long-term care; research methods

Services provided: Photocopy machine; reference; alerting/SDI; bibliography preparation; database searching by staff; interlibrary loan (borrowing only)

Automation: MEDLARS for database searching

Publications: Current Awareness for Resources in Geriatric Education (monthly)

Gerontology/geriatrics libraries organization: Yes; willing to help start

New York City

NY-3 THE ELDER CRAFTSMEN, INC. LIBRARY. 851 Lexington Avenue, New York, NY 10021. Telephone: 212-861-3777

Type: Association

Person-in-charge: Linda Cross

Staff: 1 volunteer (part-time)

Founded: 1955

Hours: Monday-Wednesday, Friday 10a.m.-5:30p.m.

Subject strengths: Adult education/creativity

Services provided: Reference

NY-4 FORDHAM UNIVERSITY. THIRD AGE CENTER. LIBRARY. 113 West 60th Street, New York, NY 10023. Telephone: 212-841-5347

Type: Academic

Person-in-charge: Melba Chamberlain

Staff: 1 paraprofessional (part-time)

Founded: 1978

Hours: Monday-Friday 9a.m.-5p.m.

Holdings: 400 monographs; 5 current serial titles

Subject strengths: Health care; long-term care; social services

NY-5 JEWISH HOME AND HOSPITAL FOR THE AGED. FREDERICK ZEMEN MEMORIAL LIBRARY. 120 West 106th Street, New York, NY 10025. Telephone: 212-870-4962. FAX: 212-870-4905

Type: Nursing home

Librarian: Yisroel Messik

Staff: 1 professional librarian (part-time)

Founded: 1942

Hours: 15 hours a week

Holdings: 900 monographs; 50 current serial titles; 3 audiocassettes; 6 microform titles

Subject strengths: Death and dying; geriatrics; health care; living arrangements; long-term care; physiology; psychology/mental health; research methods; social services

Special collections: Reprint collection of 430 titles dating from 1914

Services provided: Reference; bibliography preparation; indexing/abstracting; database searching by staff; circulation; interlibrary loan (borrowing and lending)

Automation: MARCIVE for cataloging, EBSCO for serials management; BRS, DIALOG and MEDLARS for database searching

Networks: Manhattan/Bronx Health Sciences Libraries Group.

Serial titles are listed in SERHOLD (National Library of Medicine).

Gerontology/geriatrics libraries organization: Yes; willing to help start

NY-6 NEW YORK CITY. DEPARTMENT FOR THE AGING. LIBRARY. 2 Lafayette Street, 7th floor, New York, NY 10007. Telephone: 212-577-0647. FAX: 212-587-3274

Type: Area Agency on Aging (AAA)

Librarian: Winifred Lieber

Staff: 1 professional librarian (part-time)

Founded: 1970

Hours: 11a.m.-4p.m. four days a week

Holdings: 27 current serial and newsletter titles; 1 newspaper title; 40 pamphlet file drawers

Subject strengths: Aging network; demographic/census/statistics; economic; employment; government documents; health care; living arrangements; long-term care; policy issues; retirement; social services

Special collections: Archival collection of agency publications

Services provided: Photocopy machine; reference; alerting/SDI; circulation; interlibrary loan (borrowing only); archives management

Gerontology/geriatrics libraries organization: Yes

Rochester

NY-7 MONROE COMMUNITY HOSPITAL. T. F. WILLIAMS HEALTH SCIENCES LIBRARY. 435 East Henrietta Road, Rochester, NY 14620. Telephone: 716-274-7362. FAX: 716-274-7149. OCLC code: VQU

Type: Medical

Librarian: Elinor Reynolds

Staff: 1 professional librarian; 1 volunteer (part-time)

Founded: 1970

Hours: Open 24 hours a day, 7 days a week

Holdings: 921 monographs; 186 current serial titles; 2 newspaper titles; 5 pamphlet file drawers

Subject strengths: Administration; geriatrics; health care; long-term care; social services

Services provided: Photocopy machine; reference; bibliography preparation; database searching by staff; circulation; interlibrary loan (borrowing and lending)

Automation: Microcomputer; OCLC and DOCLINE for interlibrary loan; MEDLARS and CompuServe for database searching

Networks: Rochester Regional Library Council (RRLC); Rochester Area Libraries in Health Care (RALIH).

Monograph and serial titles are listed in OCLC.

NORTH CAROLINA

Chapel Hill

NC-1 UNIVERSITY OF NORTH CAROLINA AT CHAPEL HILL. HEALTH SERVICES RESEARCH CENTER. LIBRARY. Chase Hall, Campus Box #7490, Chapel Hill, NC 27599-7490. Telephone: 919-966-7126. FAX: 919-966-5764

Type: Academic

Librarian: Lynn Whitener

Staff: 1 professional librarian, 2 assistants (part-time)

Founded: 1968

Hours: Monday-Friday 8a.m.-5p.m.

Holdings: 200 monographs; 5 current serial titles; 2 newspaper titles; 18 pamphlet file drawers

Subject strengths: Administration; demographic/census/statistics; economic; geriatrics; government documents; health care; long-term care; policy issues

Services provided: Photocopy machine; reference; alerting/SDI; bibliography preparation; indexing and abstracting; database searching by staff (fee charged for some users); circulation; AV distribution; archives management

Automation: Microcomputer; shared network/utility access to the University of North Carolina at Chapel Hill mainframe computer; BRS and MEDLARS for database searching; Microsoft Word and ProCite for word processing, bibliographic management, etc.

Gerontology/geriatrics libraries organization: Yes; willing to help start

Comment: The on-site collection is mainly a repository for hard-to-find materials; the library relies heavily on resources at other University of North Carolina libraries to fill information needs.

Durham

NC-2 DUKE UNIVERSITY MEDICAL CENTER. CENTER FOR THE STUDY OF AGING AND HUMAN DEVELOPMENT/DUKE GERIATRIC EDUCATION CENTER. LIBRARY. Duke University Medical Center, Box 3003, Durham, NC 27710. Telephone: 919-684-5826 or 684-5149. FAX: 919-684-8666

Type: Medical
Person-in-charge: Erdman Palmore
Staff: 1 paraprofessional (part-time)
Founded: 1957/1988
Hours: 40 hours a week
Holdings: 200 monographs
Subject strengths: Geriatrics

OHIO

Cleveland

OH-1 THE BENJAMIN ROSE INSTITUTE. LIBRARY. 1422 Euclid Avenue, #500, Cleveland, OH 44115. Telephone: 216-621-7201

Type: Nursing home
Librarian: Karen M. Bensing
Staff: 1 professional librarian
Founded: 1971
Hours: Monday-Friday 9a.m.-5p.m.
Holdings: 2,500 monographs; 66 current serial titles; 5

newspaper titles; 14 pamphlet file drawers

Subject strengths: Administration; aging network; demographic/census/statistics; geriatrics; living arrangements; long-term care; policy issues; psychology/mental health; research methods; social services

Special collections: Repository for the papers and publications of the Margaret Blenkner Research Institute of the Benjamin Rose Institute; complete set of the annual reports of the Institute dating back to 1909

Services provided: Photocopy machine; reference; alerting/SDI; bibliography preparation; database searching by staff; circulation; interlibrary loan (borrowing and lending); AV distribution; archives management

Automation: Microcomputer; ProCite for cataloging; BRS, DIALOG, and MEDLARS for database searching; WordPerfect for word processing, etc.

Networks: Medical Library Association of Northeast Ohio.

Serial titles are listed in a local union list of serials.

Publications: Library Current Awareness Service (monthly)

Gerontology/geriatrics libraries organization: Yes; willing to help start

OH-2 CASE WESTERN RESERVE UNIVERSITY. ELDERLY CARE RESEARCH CENTER. LIBRARY. Mather Memorial, Room 226, Cleveland, OH 44106. Telephone: 216-368-2700. FAX: 216-368-2704

Type: Academic

Person-in-charge: Eva Kahana

Staff: 3 paraprofessionals (part-time)

Founded: 1968

Hours: Monday-Friday 8:30a.m.-5p.m.

Holdings: 500 monographs; 20 current serial titles; 3 pamphlet file drawers

Subject strengths: Anthropology/ethnicity; death and dying; geriatrics; health care; social services

Services provided: Circulation; interlibrary loan (borrowing only)

Automation: Minicomputer

Columbus

OH-3 OHIO. DEPARTMENT OF AGING. RESOURCE CENTER. 50 West Broad Street, 9th floor, Columbus, OH 43266-0501. Telephone: 614-466-9086. FAX: 614-466-5741

Type: State Unit on Aging (SUA)

Librarian: Sally Brown

Staff: 1 professional librarian, 1 paraprofessional (part-time)

Founded: 1973

Hours: Monday-Friday 8a.m.-4:45p.m.

Holdings: 2,000 monographs; 90 current serial titles; 2 newspaper titles; 50 audiocassettes; 100 videocassettes; 90 16mm films; 6 pamphlet file drawers

Subject strengths: Administration; aging network; death and dying; demographic/census/statistics; economic; employment; government documents; health care; living arrangements; international; long-term care; physiology; policy issues; psychology/mental health; retirement; social services

Special collections: Annual reports and special publications of the Ohio Department of Aging

Services provided: Reference; alerting/SDI; circulation; interlibrary loan (borrowing only); AV distribution

Automation: Microcomputer; Winnebago software for cataloging, circulation, and online catalog; WordPerfect for word processing, etc.

Hamilton

OH-4 MERCY HOSPITAL. GOLDEN LIFE CARE LIBRARY. 100 Riverfront Plaza, Hamilton, OH 45011. Telephone: 513-867-6458. FAX: 513-867-1613

Type: Nursing home

Librarian: Sister Mary Annrita, R.S.M.

Staff: 1 professional librarian, 4 volunteers (part-time)

Founded: 1970

Hours: Monday-Friday 8a.m.-4:30p.m.

Holdings: 209 monographs; 14 current serial titles

Subject strengths: Administration; consumer materials; geriatrics; health care; living arrangements; social services

Services provided: Photocopy machine; reference; database searching by staff; circulation; interlibrary loan (borrowing and lending)

Automation: Microcomputer; BRS for database searching

Publications: Golden Life Care (bimonthly newsletter) has a "From the Library" column.

Comment: There are 2 separate Golden Life Care libraries at Mercy Hospital; one at Hamilton and one at Fairfield. They are administered from the Health Sciences Library at Mercy Hospital at Hamilton. The libraries are for public use by the elderly.

Oxford

OH-5 MIAMI UNIVERSITY. SCRIPPS GERONTOLOGY CENTER. LIBRARY. Oxford, OH 45056. Telephone: 513-529-2914

Type: Academic

Person-in-charge: Robert C. Atchley

Staff: 2 assistants (part-time)

Founded: 1922

Hours: Monday-Friday 8a.m.-5p.m.

Holdings: 1,000 monographs; 35 current serial titles; 3 pamphlet file drawers

Subject strengths: Administration; aging network; demographic/census/statistics; long-term care; policy issues; social services

Special collections: Archival collection from the Scripps Foundation for Research in Population Problems

Comment: Library is for use by faculty and research staff.

OREGON

OR-1 OREGON GERIATRIC EDUCATION CENTER. RESOURCE CENTER. Portland State University, P.O. Box 751, Portland, OR 97207-0751. Telephone: 503-725-5149. FAX: 503-725-5199

Type: Geriatric education center (GEC)

Librarian: Jennifer S. Gregorio

Staff: 1 professional librarian (part-time), 1 assistant (part-time)

Founded: 1989

Hours: Monday-Friday 9a.m.-5p.m.

Holdings: 100 monographs; 10 current serial titles

Subject strengths: Demographic/census/statistics; education/training; geriatrics; health care; long-term care; psychology/mental health; social services

Services provided: Photocopy machine; reference; database searching by staff (fee charged for some users); circulation; interlibrary loan (borrowing and lending)

Automation: Microcomputer; DataEase for acquisitions, cataloging, and circulation; BRS and MEDLARS for database searching

Networks: Portland Area Health Sciences Librarians; Oregon Health Sciences Libraries Association

Publications: GeriTRACS (quarterly newsletter of the Oregon Geriatric Education Center) has a "Resources" column.

Gerontology/geriatrics libraries organization: Yes; willing to help start

Comment: The Oregon Geriatric Education Center has 3 participating institutions: the Oregon Health Sciences University in Portland (location of the main GEC office); the Portland State University, Institute on Aging (location of the administration of the GEC resource center); and the Portland Veterans Administration Center.

PENNSYLVANIA

Lima

PA-1 FAIR ACRES GERIATRIC CENTER. MEDICAL

LIBRARY. Route 352, Lima, PA 19037. Telephone: 215-891-5717
Type: Nursing home
Person-in-charge: Lisa A. Maffei
Staff: 1 paraprofessional (part-time)
Founded: 1980
Hours: Monday-Friday 8:30a.m.-4:30p.m.
Holdings: 100 monographs; 15 current serial titles
Subject strengths: Administration; aging network; health care; long-term care; physiology; psychology/mental health
Services provided: Photocopy machine; reference; alerting/SDI; interlibrary loan (borrowing and lending)
Networks: Consortium for Health Information and Library Services (CHI)

Philadelphia

PA-2 PHILADELPHIA CORPORATION FOR AGING. LIBRARY. 642 North Broad Street, Philadelphia, PA 19130-3409. Telephone: 215-765-9000. FAX: 215-765-9066
Type: Area Agency on Aging (AAA)
Librarian: Maureen Neville
Staff: 1 professional librarian, 1 paraprofessional (part-time)
Founded: 1978
Hours: Monday-Friday 9a.m.-5p.m.
Holdings: 1,900 monographs; 39 current serial titles; 40 newsletter titles; 11 microform titles; 16 pamphlet file drawers
Subject strengths: Aging network; demographic/census/statistics; economic; employment; geriatrics;

health care; living arrangements; long-term care; policy issues; psychology/mental health; social services

Special collections: Channeling demonstration publications; Philadelphia Corporation for Aging archives including contracts awarded to providers of services to the aged in Philadelphia; Pennsylvania Department of Aging and City of Philadelphia publications on aging; SCAN microfiche collection

Services provided: Reference; alerting/SDI; bibliography preparation; database searching by staff; circulation; interlibrary loan (borrowing and lending)

Automation: BRS for database searching; agency shared network/utility system for word processing, etc.

Networks: National Library of Medicine Regional Medical Library Network

Publications: Acquisition List (quarterly)

Gerontology/geriatrics libraries organization: Willing to help start

PA-3 PHILADELPHIA GERIATRIC CENTER. LIBRARY. 5301 Old York Road, Philadelphia, PA 19141. Telephone: 215-456-2971 or 456-2001. FAX: 215-456-2017

Type: Nursing home

Librarian: Joyce A. Post

Staff: 1 professional librarian, 1 assistant (part-time), 1 volunteer (part-time)

Founded: 1959

Hours: Monday-Friday 9a.m.-5p.m. (accessible at other hours by staff)

Holdings: 11,000 monographs; 205 current serial titles; 1 pamphlet file drawer

Subject strengths: Administration; anthropology/ethnicity; death and dying; demographic/census/statistics; economic; geriatrics; health care; living arrangements; international; long-term care; policy issues; psychology/mental health; research methods; social services

Special collections: Papers of Elaine Brody

Services provided: Photocopy machine; reference; bibliography preparation; database searching by staff (fee charged for some users); circulation; interlibrary loan (borrowing and lending; fee charged for some users)

Automation: Microcomputer; Baker & Taylor's Link for acquisitions; Librarian's Helper for cataloging; DBase for serials management; BRS and MEDLARS for database searching; DOCLINE for interlibrary loan; ProCite for bibliographic management; Wordstar for word processing, etc.

Networks: Delaware Valley Information Consortium (DEVIC); National Library of Medicine Regional Medical Library Network; Basic Health Sciences Libraries Group (BHSL); Pennsylvania Regional Interlibrary Loan Group (PRILL).

Serial titles are listed in SERHOLD (National Library of Medicine).

Publications: Newsletter/Acquisitions list (bimonthly)

Gerontology/geriatrics libraries organization: Yes; willing to help start

Comment: There are 2 separate professional libraries: a research library and a medical library. There is also a residents' library of 300 volumes for which the library acts as a technical consultant.

PA-4 TEMPLE UNIVERSITY. INSTITUTE ON AGING. RESOURCE CENTER. 1601 North Broad Street, Philadelphia, PA 19122. Telephone: 215-787-3208

Type: Academic
Person-in-charge: Kathy Segrist
Staff: 1 paraprofessional (part-time)
Founded: 1978
Hours: Monday-Friday 8:30a.m.-4:30p.m.
Holdings: Number of monographs is unknown; 11 current serial titles; 2 audiocassettes; 10 videocassettes; 1,000 microform titles; 25 pamphlet file drawers
Subject strengths: Administration; aging network; demographic/census/statistics; economic; geriatrics; government documents; health care; long-term care; research methods; social services
Special collections: SCAN microfiche collection
Services provided: Photocopy machine; reference; database searching by staff (fee charged for all users); archives management
Automation: BRS and DIALOG for database searching
Gerontology/geriatrics libraries organization: Yes; willing to help start
Comment: Coadministers, with the University of Pittsburgh, the Geriatric Education Center of Pennsylvania.

PA-5 UNIVERSITY OF PENNSYLVANIA. CENTER FOR AGING. LIBRARY. 3615 Chestnut Street, Philadelphia, PA 19104. Telephone: 215-898-3163. FAX: 215-898-0580
Type: Academic
Person-in-charge: Nancy Ellis
Staff: 1 assistant (part-time)
Founded: 1978
Hours: Monday-Friday 9a.m.-5p.m.
Holdings: 6 current serial titles; 10 audiocassettes; 7

videocassettes
Subject strengths: Aging network; demographic/census/statistics; economic; government documents; policy issues
Services provided: Circulation

University Park

PA-6 THE PENNSYLVANIA STATE UNIVERSITY. HUMAN DEVELOPMENT WORKING COLLECTION. S-109 Human Development Building, University Park, PA 16802. Telephone: 814-863-0776
Type: Academic
Librarian: Fay C. Wohlwill
Staff: 1 professional librarian (part-time), 1 assistant (part-time)
Founded: 1973
Hours: Monday-Friday 9a.m.-5p.m.
Holdings: 3,000 monographs; 30 current serial titles; 40 pamphlet file drawers; 720 Ph.D and Masters theses
Subject strengths: Psychology/mental health; social services
Services provided: Photocopy machine; reference; alerting/SDI; bibliography preparation; circulation
Automation: Microcomputer; PsycLIT on SilverPlatter is accessed at the main university library
Gerontology/geriatrics libraries organization: Yes; willing to help start
Comment: Began as a gerontology collection that is now expanded to include child, adolescent, family, and life-span material.

RHODE ISLAND

RI-1 RHODE ISLAND. DEPARTMENT OF ELDERLY AFFAIRS. EVE M. GOLDBERG LIBRARY AND RESOURCE CENTER. 79 Washington Street, Providence, RI 02903. Telephone: 401-277-2880

Type: State Unit on Aging and Area Agency on Aging (SUA/AAA)

Person-in-charge: Will Speck

Staff: 1 paraprofessional (part-time), 1 assistant (part-time)

Founded: 1958

Hours: Monday-Friday 8:30a.m.-4p.m.

Holdings: 500 monographs; 15 current serial titles; 15 newsletter titles; 50 videocassettes; 6 pamphlet file drawers

Subject strengths: Economic; health care; living arrangements; retirement; social services

Services provided: Reference; alerting/SDI; circulation; AV distribution

TENNESSEE

TN-1 TENNESSEE. COMMISSION ON AGING. LIBRARY. 706 Church Street, Suite 201, Nashville, TN 37243-0860. Telephone: 615-741-2056

Type: State Unit on Aging (SUA)

Person-in-charge: Steve Canada or Mason Rowe

Staff: 2 paraprofessionals (part-time)

Founded: 1963

Hours: Monday-Friday 8a.m.-4:30p.m.

Holdings: 500 monographs; 10 current serial titles; 54 videocassettes; 16 pamphlet file drawers; 42 slide presentations; 39 films

Subject strengths: Aging network; demographic/census/statistics; long-term care; planning/program development; policy issues; social services

Special collections: Early minutes and manuscripts from the Tennessee Commission on Aging

Services provided: Photocopy machine; reference; database searching by staff; AV distribution

Automation: Microcomputer

Networks: State Government Libraries in Tennessee. Titles are listed with the Tennessee State Library system and with the special libraries in Tennessee State Government.

TEXAS

Austin

TX-1 TEXAS. DEPARTMENT ON AGING. RESOURCE LIBRARY. P.O. Box 12786, Capitol Station, South Austin, TX 78711-3702. Telephone: 512-444-2727. FAX: 512-440-5290

Type: State Unit on Aging (SUA)

Person-in-charge: Paula Johnson

Founded: 1972

Hours: Monday-Friday 8a.m.-5p.m.

Holdings: 5 current serial titles; 15 audiocassettes; 65 videocassettes

Subject strengths: Administration; aging network; consumer materials; government documents;

Services provided: Photocopy machine; reference; AV distribution

Comment: Library is for office staff and service providers.

Denton

TX-2 UNIVERSITY OF NORTH TEXAS. LIBRARIES. MEDIA LIBRARY. GERONTOLOGICAL FILM COLLECTION. P.O. Box 12898, Denton, TX 76203. Telephone: 817-565-2489

Type: Academic

Librarian: George D. Mitchell

Staff: 1 professional librarian (part-time), 1 paraprofessional (part-time), 1 assistant

Founded: 1971

Hours: Monday-Friday 8a.m.-5p.m.; hours vary according to the academic year

Holdings: 12 videocassettes; 300 16 mm films

Subject strengths: Administration; anthropology/ethnicity; death and dying; films; geriatrics; health care; living arrangements; long-term care; social services

Services provided: 16mm projectors; sound/slide projectors; reference (films only); bibliography preparation; AV distribution

Automation: Microcomputer; cataloging, circulation, and online catalog available through shared network/utility system of main university library; OCLC for interlibrary loan; Media Minder for booking of films

Networks: OCLC; Association for Higher Education of North Texas Area; Consortium of College and University Media Centers.

Film titles are listed in the the Association for High er Education of North Texas Area Union List of Media and in the Educational Film and Video Locator (published by R.R. Bowker).

Publications: Printed catalog of holdings (updated annually)

Comment: Films are selected by the faculty of the University of North Texas Studies in Aging program. Films are lent throughout the United States.

San Antonio

TX-3 SOUTH TEXAS GERIATRIC EDUCATION CENTER. LIBRARY/RESOURCE CENTER. University of Texas Health Science Center (UTHSC) at San Antonio. 7703 Floyd Curl Drive, San Antonio, TX 78284-7919. Telephone: 512-567-3370

Type: Geriatric education center (GEC)

Person-in-charge: Carolyn Marshall

Staff: 1 paraprofessional (part-time), 1 assistant (part-time)

Founded: 1985

Hours: Monday-Friday 8a.m.-5p.m.

Holdings: 50 monographs; 6 audiocassettes; 200 videocassettes

Subject strengths: Demographic/census/statistics; economic; geriatrics; long-term care

Services provided: Circulation; interlibrary loan (lending only); AV distribution

Comment: Uses the resources of the libraries at the UTHSC at San Antonio and the Audie L. Murphy Memorial Veterans Hospital (ALMMVH) in addition to its own collection.

VIRGINIA

VA-1 AMERICAN COLLEGE OF HEALTH CARE ADMINISTRATORS. LIBRARY. 325 South Patrick Street, Alexandria, VA 22314. Telephone: 703-549-

5822. FAX: 703-739-7901
Type: Association
Librarian: Doris K. Mela
Staff: 1 professional librarian (part-time)
Founded: 1962
Hours: Open 20 hours a week
Holdings: Number of monographs unknown at the time of the survey; 90 current serial titles; 6 audiocassettes; 15 pamphlet file drawers
Subject strengths: Administration; aging network; economic; government documents; long-term care
Services provided: Photocopy machine; reference; bibliography preparation; circulation; interlibrary loan (borrowing and lending)
Automation: Microcomputer
Comment: Membership in the association consists of persons engaged in the administration of long-term care facilities or interested in nursing home and long-term care administration. Formerly called the American College of Nursing Home Administrators.

WASHINGTON

Seattle

WA-1 NATIONAL PACIFIC/ASIAN RESOURCE CENTER ON AGING. 1511 Third Avenue, Suite 914, Seattle, WA 98101. Telephone: 206-624-1221
Type: National resource center (NRC)
Person-in-charge: Brian Fujimoto
Staff: 3 paraprofessionals (part-time), 2 assistants (part-time)
Founded: 1979

Hours: Monday-Friday 8:30a.m.-5p.m.
Holdings: 250 monograph titles; 10 current serial titles
Subject strengths: Anthropology/ethnicity; demographic/census/statistics; government documents; policy issues; social services
Services provided: Photocopy machine; reference
Automation: Microcomputer; word processing, etc.

WA-2 NORTHWEST GERIATRIC CLEARINGHOUSE. RESOURCE CENTER. University of Washington, HL-23, Seattle, WA 98195. Telephone: 206-685-7478. FAX: 206-685-3436
Type: Geriatric education center (GEC)
Person-in-charge: Susan Guralnick
Staff: 1 paraprofessional (part-time), 1 assistant (part-time)
Founded: 1985
Hours: Monday-Friday 8a.m.-5p.m.
Holdings: 600 monographs; 10 current serial titles; 15 newsletter titles; 90 videocassettes
Subject strengths: Economic; geriatrics; long-term care; policy issues; social services
Services provided: Photocopy machine; reference; alerting/SDI; circulation

WEST VIRGINIA

WV-1 WEST VIRGINIA. STATE COMMISSION ON AGING. LIBRARY. State Capitol, Charleston, WV 25305. Telephone: 304-348-2917
Type: State Unit on Aging (SUA)
Person-in-charge: Tom Dudley
Staff: 1 paraprofessional (part-time)
Founded: 1972

Hours: Monday-Friday 7:30a.m.-3:30p.m.

Holdings: 5,000 monographs; 25 current serial titles; 50 videocassettes

Subject strengths: Administration; demographic/census/statistics; economic; policy issues; social services

Services provided: Reference; alerting/SDI; circulation; interlibrary loan (borrowing only); AV distribution

PUERTO RICO

PR-1 GERIATRIC EDUCATION CENTER OF THE UNIVERSITY OF PUERTO RICO SCHOOL OF MEDICINE. RESOURCE UNIT. G. P. O. Box 5067, San Juan, PR 00936. Telephone: 809-751-2478. FAX: 809-765-0514

Type: Geriatric education center (GEC)

Person-in-charge: Carmen Ana Suarez

Staff: 2 paraprofessionals (part-time), 2 assistants (part-time)

Founded: 1985

Hours: Monday-Friday 8a.m.-5p.m.

Holdings: 200 monographs; 8 current serial titles; 120 videocassettes; 3 pamphlet file drawers

Subject strengths: Death and dying; geriatrics; health care; living arrangements; research methods; social services

Services provided: Photocopy machine; reference; AV distribution

Automation: Microcomputer; word processing, etc.

CANADA

British Columbia

CAN-1 SIMON FRASER UNIVERSITY. GERONTOLOGY RESEARCH CENTRE. INFORMATION CENTRE. 515 West Hastings Street, Vancouver, British Columbia, Canada V6B 5K3. Telephone: 604-291-5064. FAX: 604-291-5066

Type: Academic

Librarian: Janet Heekin

Staff: 1 professional librarian

Founded: 1982

Hours: Monday-Friday 9a.m.-4:30p.m.

Holdings: 5,000 monographs; 9 current serial titles; 15 newspaper titles; 30 audiocassettes; 10 videocassettes; 7 pamphlet file drawers; reprint file of 10,000 articles

Subject strengths: Aging network; demographic/census/statistics; government documents; health care; living arrangements; long-term care

Services provided: Photocopy machine; reference; alerting/SDI; bibliography preparation; database searching by staff (fee charged some users); AV distribution

Automation: Microcomputer; DIALOG for database searching

Gerontology/geriatrics libraries organization: Yes; willing to help start

Manitoba

CAN-2 BETHANIA MENNONITE PERSONAL CARE HOME. LIBRARY. 1045 Concordia Avenue, Winnipeg, Manitoba, Canada R2K 3S7. Telephone: 204-667-0795. FAX: 204-667-7078

Type: Nursing home

Person-in-charge: Esther Fransen

Staff: 1 paraprofessional (part-time)

Founded: 1960

Hours: Monday-Friday 8:30a.m.-4:30p.m.

Holdings: 512 monographs; 24 current serial titles; 24 audiocassettes; 12 videocassettes

Subject strengths: Administration; geriatrics; health care; long-term care

Services provided: Photocopy machine; alerting/SDI, circulation; interlibrary loan (borrowing only)

Networks: Manitoba Health Libraries Association

CAN-3 J. W. CRANE MEMORIAL LIBRARY. Deer Lodge Centre, 2109 Portage Avenue, Winnipeg, Manitoba, Canada R3E 0W3. Telephone: 204-831-2152. FAX: 204-888-5574

Type: Nursing home

Librarian: Judy Inglis

Staff: 1 professional librarian, 2 paraprofessionals (part-time), 4 volunteers (part-time)

Founded: 1983

Hours: Monday-Friday 9a.m.-4:30p.m.

Holdings: 4,000 monographs; 185 current serial titles; 3 CD-ROM titles; 2 pamphlet file drawers

Subject strengths: Administration; geriatrics; government documents (Canadian); health care; long-term care; social services

Special collections: University Microfilms International microfiche collection in gerontology and geriatrics

Services provided: Photocopy machine; reference; alerting/SDI; bibliography preparation; indexing and abstracting; database searching by staff (fee charged some users); circulation; interlibrary loan (borrowing and lending; fee charged some users); AV distribution

Automation: Microcomputer; INMAGIC for cataloging; BRS and SilverPlatter for database searching; WordPerfect for word processing, etc.

Networks: Serial titles listed in the Manitoba Health Libraries Association Union List

Publications: AgeLit (monthly); Special Bibliography Series (monthly); video catalog (annually with updates)

Gerontology/geriatrics libraries organization: Yes; willing to help start

Comment: Formerly the Deer Lodge Resource Centre in Gerontology and Geriatrics. In 1990 the J. W. Crane Library of the Canadian Geriatrics Research Society, established in 1962 and located in Toronto, Ontario, was merged with the Deer Lodge Resource Center making this combined library now the de facto national library on aging of Canada.

Ontario

CAN-4 BAYCREST CENTRE FOR GERIATRIC CARE. STAFF LIBRARY. 3560 Bathurst Street, Toronto, Ontario, Canada M6A 2E1. Telephone: 416-789-5131. FAX: 416-785-2378

Type: Nursing home
Librarian: Madeline Grant
Staff: 1 professional librarian; 1 paraprofessional; 3 volunteers (part-time)
Founded: 1982
Hours: Monday-Friday 9a.m.-5p.m.
Holdings: 2,000 monographs; 150 current serial titles; 1 newspaper title; 300 audiocassettes; 50 videocassettes; 30 pamphlet file drawers
Subject strengths: Administration; death and dying; geriatrics; health care; long-term care; physiology; psychology/mental health
Services provided: Photocopy machine; reference; alerting/SDI; bibliography preparation; database searching by staff (fee charged some users); circulation; interlibrary loan (borrowing and lending); AV distribution
Automation: Microcomputer; Sydney for acquisitions, cataloging, serials management, circulation and online catalog; BRS, DIALOG, and MEDLARS for database searching; WordPerfect, DBase and Lotus for word processing, etc.
Networks: Serial titles are listed in the Toronto Health Libraries Association Union List
Publications: New Acquisitions (3 times a year); List of Journals and Newsletters (annual); Catalog of Videocassettes
Gerontology/geriatrics libraries organization: Yes; willing to help start

Quebec

CAN-5 MAIMONIDES HOSPITAL. GERIATRIC CENTRE. POLLACK LIBRARY. 5795 Caldwell Avenue, Montreal, Quebec, Canada H4W 1W3. Telephone: 514-483-2121. FAX: 514-483-1561

Type: Medical

Person-in-charge: Sheindel Bresinger

Staff: 1 paraprofessional, 1 assistant (part-time)

Founded: 1965

Hours: Monday-Friday 8:30a.m.-4:30p.m.

Holdings: 2,089 monographs; 109 current serial titles; 1 newspaper title; 16 audiocassettes; 146 videocassettes; 4 pamphlet file drawers

Subject strengths: Administration; anthropology/ethnicity; geriatrics; long-term care; psychology/mental health; social services

Services provided: Photocopy machine; reference; alerting/SDI; bibliography preparation; database searching by staff; circulation; interlibrary loan (borrowing and lending; fee charged some users); AV distribution; archives management

Automation: Microcomputer; BRS for database searching

Networks: Serial titles are listed in the Montreal Health Libraries Association Union List

Gerontology/geriatrics libraries organization: Yes; willing to help start

Appendix A

Questionnaire

GERONTOLOGY AND GERIATRICS LIBRARIES IN THE UNITED STATES AND CANADA

A SURVEY

I. GENERAL INFORMATION

a. Library name: ______________________________

b. Institution name: ______________________________

c. Address: ______________________________

d. Name of person in charge of the library: ______________________________

e. Phone number: ( ) ______________________________

f. Fax number: ( ) ______________________________

g. E-mail number(s): ______________________________

I. GENERAL INFORMATION (continued):

h. OCLC code: ______________________________

i. Type of library (circle one):

1. Academic
2. Medical/Hospital
3. Professional association
4. Public
5. Service agency
6. Special (specify): ______________________
7. Other (specify): ______________________

II. FACILITY

a. What hours a week is the library open? __________

b. How many square feet of space does the library occupy?

____

c. What is the user seating capacity of the library?

____

d. What equipment do you have? (circle all that apply)

1. Photocopy machine
2. Reader/printer
3. Microcomputer
4. Minicomputer
5. Mainframe computer
6. CD-ROM player
7. Audiovideo equipment

II. FACILITY (continued):

8. Telefacsimile machine
9. Other: ____________________

e. Which of the following library functions are automated, either through stand-alone or integrated systems or a utility (e.g.: Librarian's Helper, ProCite, Baker & Taylor's Link, Geac, OCLC, DOCLINE, etc.)? What specific software do you use in each application?

1. Acquisitions ____________________
2. Cataloging ____________________
3. Serials ____________________
4. Circulation ____________________
5. Online public access catalog ____________________
6. Database searching ____________________
7. Interlibrary loan ____________________
8. Library administration (word processing, budgets, etc.) ____________________
9. Other: ____________________

f. Do you anticipate obtaining additional equipment or electronic hardware or software in the future? Please describe specific types and intended applications.

____
____
____

III. PERSONNEL

a. How many people work in the library? (please give numbers)

III. PERSONNEL (continued):

	Full-time	Part-time
1. Professional librarians	____	____
2. Paraprofessionals	____	____
3. Clerical/student assistants	____	____
4. Volunteers	____	____

b. What is the title of the person in charge of the library?

____

c. How many years has he/she been in this position?

____

d. What is his/her highest professional degree?

____

e. What are the titles of the other professional librarians on the staff? ____________________________

____

IV. COLLECTION

a. How many of the following types of materials does the library have?

	Total	Number added in 1989
1. Monograph titles	________	________

IV. COLLECTION (continued):

2. Journal titles (total) _____ _____
3. Journal titles (currently received only) _____ _____
4. Newspaper titles _____ _____
5. Audio cassettes _____ _____
6. Video cassettes _____ _____
7. Microfilm/fiche titles _____ _____
8. CD-ROM titles _____ _____
9. Locally mounted databases _____ _____
10. Vertical file drawers _____ _____
11. Other: _____________ _____ _____

b. Which of the following serials do you currently receive on a regular basis? (circle all that apply)

1. Age and Ageing
2. Annual Review of Gerontology and Geriatrics
3. Experimental Aging Research
4. Clinics in Geriatric Medicine
5. Generations
6. Gerontologist
7. Gerontology
8. International Journal of Aging and Human Development

IV. COLLECTION (continued):

9. Journal of Aging and Social Policy
10. Journal of the American Geriatrics Society
11. Journal of Cross-Cultural Gerontology
12. Journals of Gerontology
13. Mechanisms of Ageing and Development
14. Neurobiology of Aging
15. Older Americans Report
16. Provider
17. Psychology and Aging
18. Research on Aging

c. What are the major subject strengths of your collection? (circle all that apply)

1. Administration (retirement, nursing home, other facilities, etc.)
2. Aging network reports and documents (federal, state, local)
3. Anthropology, ethnicity, cross-cultural studies
4. Consumer materials (easy-to-read, large-print, etc.)
5. Death and dying
6. Demographic, census, statistical data, etc.
7. Economic aspects (Medicare/Medicaid, insurance, social security, business, financial, legal, etc.)
8. Employment
9. Geriatrics (medicine, nursing, rehabilitation, etc.)
10. Government documents (federal, state, local, international, etc.)
11. Health care
12. Housing, living arrangements, environmental and product design, etc.
13. International material
14. Long term care

IV. COLLECTION (continued):

15. Physiology, molecular biology, aging process, etc.
16. Policy issues
17. Psychology, psychiatry, mental health, etc.
18. Research methods, statistical methods, etc.
19. Retirement
20. Social aspects (caregiving, social services, family issues, etc.)
21. Other: ______________________________

d. Do you have any special, historical, or archival collections? (circle one)

1. No
2. Yes. Please describe these (name, subject, accessibility, etc.) in full. (Use the back of this page if you need more space) ______________________
____
____
____

e. What parts of the collection are cataloged? (circle all that apply)

1. Books
2. Journals
3. Other: ______________________________

f. What classification system(s) do you use? (circle all that apply)

1. Library of Congress
2. Dewey
3. National Library of Medicine

IV. COLLECTION (continued):

4. Other: ______________________________

g. What subject authority list(s) do you use? (circle all that apply)

1. Library of Congress
2. Sears
3. Medical Subject Headings (MeSH)
4. AgeLine thesaurus
5. Other thesaurus (specify): ________________
6. Other: ______________________________

h. Are the library holdings listed in any union list? (circle all that apply)

1. Monographs. Which lists(s)? ______________
2. Journals. Which list(s)? ________________
3. Other: ______________________________

V. SERVICES

a. What services does the library provide? (circle all that apply)

1. Reference
2. User education (bibliographic instruction)
3. Literature alerting services (current awareness, SDI, etc.)
4. Bibliography preparation
5. Indexing, abstracting
6. Database searching (by staff)
7. Database searching (by end-users)

V. SERVICES (continued):

8. End-user training
9. Microcomputer/Local area network center
10. Electronic gateway/E-mail/fax center
11. Circulation
12. Interlibrary lending
13. Interlibrary borrowing
14. Audiovisual distribution
15. Learning resource center
16. Archives management, preservation/conservation
17. Centralized purchasing
18. Other: ______________________________

b. How many reference questions were answered in March 1990? ______________________________
in 1989? ______________________________

c. What are the most frequent types of questions the library is asked? ______________________________
____
____

d. Please rank the most frequently used databases: (7 = most heavily used, 6 = next most heavily used, etc. 0 = not used)

1. ABI/Inform ____
2. AgeLine ____
3. Health Planning and Administration ____
4. MEDLINE ____
5. PsycINFO ____
6. Sociological Abstracts ____
7. Other: ______________________ ____
______________________ ____

V. SERVICES (continued):

e. Which vendors do you use? (circle all that apply)

1. BRS
2. DIALOG
3. National Library of Medicine
4. Mead Data Central
5. H. W. Wilson Co.
6. CompuServe
7. Other: ______________________________

f. Do you charge for database searches? (circle one)

1. All users
2. Some users
3. No users

g. How many database searches were completed:

	in March 1990	in 1989
1. by staff	______	______
2. by end users	______	______

h. What are the most frequent kinds of topics searched?
____
____

i. Do you provide access to any of the numerical data archives of gerontology research results? (circle one)

1. No
2. Yes. Please list the ones used and the means of ac-

V. SERVICES (continued):

cess: ______________________________
____
____

j. What reference sources and information products in gerontology and geriatrics would you like to see produced or published? How would they make your job easier?
____
____
____

k. How many items were circulated
in March 1990? ______________________________
in 1989? ______________________________

l. How many interlibrary loan items were requested from other libraries in March 1990? ______________________________
in 1989? ______________________________

m. How many interlibrary loan items were supplied to other libraries in March 1990? ______________________________
in 1989? ______________________________

n. Do you charge for interlibrary loans? (circle one)

1. All users
2. Some users
3. No users

o. What are the biggest challenges in providing service at your library? ______________________________
____
____

VI. USERS

a. Please rank your library users by amount of use (11 = heaviest user group, 10 = next highest group of users, etc. 0 = does not use the library)

1. Administrators _____
2. Business users _____
3. General public _____
4. Media _____
5. Medical personnel _____
6. Public officials _____
7. Research personnel _____
8. Service providers _____
9. Staff only _____
10. Students _____
11. Other: ______________________ _____

b. What are the biggest challenges in meeting the needs of your users? ______________________________

____

____

____

VII. NETWORKING AND MEMBERSHIPS

a. List all the national, regional, and local consortia of which the library is a member. Please spell out all acronyms. ______________________________

____

____

____

b. If you use E-mail how much of an impact does it have

VII. NETWORKING AND MEMBERSHIPS (continued):

on library operations and communications. Which functions does it simplify, complicate, etc.? ________
____
____
____

c. Name the professional organizations (library, gerontology/geriatrics, medical/health, psychological, sociological, community, other) in which the library holds memberships: ______________________________
____
____
____

d. Should there be an association of gerontology/geriatrics libraries and librarians? What should its starting activities and goals be? ______________________________
____
____

e. Would you be willing to work to form such an association? (circle one)

1. Yes
2. No

VIII. PUBLIC RELATIONS

a. Do you use any public relations or marketing techniques to publicize the library? (circle one)

1. Yes. Which ones are particularly effective?

VIII. PUBLIC RELATIONS (continued):

____

____

____

2. No. Reason(s) ____________________________

b. Do you issue any publications? List the title and frequency of each: ____________________________

____

____

Would you please return a copy of the latest issue of each title with this questionnaire?

IX. ADDITIONAL COMMENTS

Please use the space below for additional comments about the topics covered in this survey and how they impact on your library functions and services.

Appendix B

Types of Libraries and Collections

ACADEMIC INSTITUTIONS

Boston University. Gerontology Center. Louis Lowy Library in Gerontology (MA-1)

Case Western Reserve University. Elderly Care Research Center. Library (OH-2)

Fordham University. Third Age Center. Library (NY-4)

Kansas State University. Center for Aging. Gerontology Library (KS-1)

Miami University. Scripps Gerontology Center. Library (OH-5)

Pennsylvania State University. Human Development Working Collection (PA-6)

Simon Fraser University. Gerontology Research Centre. Information Centre (CAN-1)

Temple University. Institute on Aging. Resource Center (PA-4)

University of California. San Francisco. Institute for Health and Aging. Resource Center (CA-5)

University of Connecticut Geriatric Education Center. Travelers Center on Aging. Education Resource Center (CT-1)

University of Florida. Center for Gerontological Studies. Reference Library (FL-1)

University of Missouri-Columbia. Social and Behavioral Sciences Reference Center (MO-1)
University of Nebraska at Omaha. Department of Gerontology. Private department collection (NE-1)
University of North Carolina at Chapel Hill. Health Services Research Center. Library (NC-1)
University of North Texas. Libraries. Media Library. Gerontological Film Collection (TX-2)
University of Pennsylvania. Center for Aging. Library (PA-5)
University of South Florida. Suncoast Gerontology Center. Eastern Star Library on Alzheimer's Disease (FL-4)
University of Southern California. Andrus Gerontology Center. Andrus Gerontology Library (CA-4)
University of West Florida. Center on Aging (FL-3)

ASSOCIATIONS

American Association of Retired Persons. Research Information Center (DC-1)
American College of Health Care Administrators. Library (VA-1)
Asociacion Nacional Pro Personas Mayores. Library (CA-3)
Center for Social Gerontology, Inc. Library (MI-1)
Center for the Study of Aging. Library (NY-1)
Elder Craftsmen, Inc. Library (NY-3)
National Alliance of Senior Citizens. Library (DC-3)
National Council on the Aging, Inc. Ollie A. Randall Library (DC-4)

National Council of Senior Citizens. Information Center (DC-5)

GERIATRIC EDUCATION CENTERS

Geriatric Education Center of the University of Puerto Rico School of Medicine. Resource Unit (PR-1)
Great Lakes Geriatric Education Center. Resource Center (IL-2)
Northwest Geriatric Clearinghouse. Resource Center (WA-2)
Ohio Valley Appalachia Regional Geriatric Education Center (KY-1)
Oregon Geriatric Education Center. Resource Center (OR-1)
Pacific Islands Geriatric Education Center. Reference Library (HI-1)
South Texas Geriatric Education Center. Library/Resource Center (TX-3)
Western New York Geriatric Education Center. Resource Center (NY-2)

GOVERNMENT

Minnesota. Department of Human Services. Library (MN-1)
Social Security Administration. Library (MD-2)
Social Security Administration. District of Columbia Branch Library (DC-6)

HOSPITALS, NURSING HOMES, MEDICAL CENTERS

Alta Bates-Herrick Hospital. Vintage Health Library and Resource Center (CA-1)

Baycrest Centre for Geriatric Care. Staff Library (CAN-4)

Benjamin Rose Institute. Library (OH-1)

Bethania Mennonite Personal Care Home. Library (CAN-2)

J. W. Crane Memorial Library (CAN-3)

Duke University Medical Center. Center for the Study of Aging and Human Development/Duke Geriatric Education Center. Library (NC-2)

Fair Acres Geriatric Center. Medical Library (PA-1)

Hartford Hospital. Jefferson House. Gerontology Resource Center (CT-2)

Jewish Home and Hospital for the Aged. Frederick Zemen Memorial Library (NY-5)

Maimonides Hospital. Geriatric Centre. Pollack Library (CAN-5)

Mercy Hospital. Golden Life Care Library (OH-4)

Monroe Community Hospital. T. F. Williams Health Sciences Library (NY-7)

Philadelphia Geriatric Center. Library (PA-3)

University of Miami School of Medicine. Center for Adult Development and Aging/Miami Area Geriatric Education Center. U. M. Pomerance Library and Resource Center (FL-2)

NATIONAL RESOURCE CENTERS

American Association of Retired Persons. National Resource Center on Health Promotion and Aging (DC-2)

Brandeis University. Heller Graduate School. Health Policy Center. Library (MA-3)

National Pacific/Asian Resource Center on Aging (WA-1)

RESEARCH CENTERS

Age Wave, Inc. Library (CA-2)
Herman Miller Research Corporation. Library (MI-2)
National Institute on Aging. Gerontolology Research Center Library (MD-1)
USDA Human Nutrition Research Center on Aging at Tufts University. Library (MA-2)

STATE UNITS ON AGING/AREA AGENCIES ON AGING

Area Agency on Aging of Western Michigan, Inc. Reference and Audiovisual Library (MI-4)
Delaware. Division of Aging. Library (DE-1)
Detroit Area Agency on Aging. Library (MI-3)
City of Chicago. Department on Aging and Disability. Library (IL-1)
New York City. Department for the Aging. Library (NY-6)
Ohio. Department of Aging. Resource Center (OH-3)
Philadelphia Corporation for Aging. Library (PA-2)
Pima Council on Aging. Resource Library (AZ-1)
Region 1-B Area Agency on Aging. Library (MI-5)
Rhode Island. Department of Elderly Affairs. Eve M. Goldberg Library and Resource Center (RI-1)
Tennessee. Commission on Aging. Library (TN-1)
Texas. Department on Aging. Resource Library (TX-1)
West Virginia. State Commission on Aging. Library (WV-1)

Appendix C

Selected Serial Holdings

AGE AND AGING — CA-3, CA-4, CT-1, CT-2, DC-1, HI-1, MD-1, MI-3, NY-3, NY-7, OH-2, PA-3, WV-1, CAN-3, CAN-4, CAN-5

ANNUAL REVIEW OF GERONTOLOGY AND GERIATRICS — CA-1, CA-4, CA-5, CT-2, DC-1, DC-4, FL-2, HI-1, MD-1, MD-2, MA-2, NY-7, PA-3, PA-6, WV-1, CAN-2, CAN-3, CAN-4, CAN-5

EXPERIMENTAL AGING RESEARCH — CA-4, CT-1, DC-1, DC-4, MD-1, PA-3, PA-6, CAN-3

CLINICS IN GERIATRIC MEDICINE — CT-1, CT-2, DC-4, FL-2, HI-1, MD-1, MN-1, NY-5, NY-7, PA-3, WV-1, CAN-3, CAN-4, CAN-5

GENERATIONS — AZ-1, CA-1, CA-2, CA-3, CA-4, CA-5, CT-2, DC-1, DC-2, DC-4, FL-1, FL-2, HI-1, IL-1, MD-1, MD-2, MA-1, MA-3, MI-1, MI-2, MI-3, MI-4, MI-5, MN-1, NE-1, NY-4, NY-6, NY-7, OH-1, OH-3, OH-5, PA-2, PA-3, PA-4, PA-5, PA-6, WA-1, WA-2, WV-1, CAN-4, CAN-5

GERONTOLOGIST — AZ-1, CA-1, CA-2, CA-3, CA-4, CA-5, CT-2, DE-1, DC-1, DC-4, DC-6, FL-1, FL-2, FL-3, HI-1, IL-1, MD-1, MD-2, MA-1, MA-3, MI-1, MI-2, MI-3, MI-4, MI-5, MN-1, MO-1, NE-1, NY-1, NY-2, NY-4, NY-5, NY-6, NY-7, NC-1, OH-1, OH-2, OH-3, OH-4, OH-5, OR-1, PA-2, PA-3, PA-5, PA-6, RI-1, TN-1, VA-1, WA-1, WA-2, WV-1, PR-1, CAN-1, CAN-2, CAN-3, CAN-4, CAN-5

GERONTOLOGY — CA-1, CA-3, CA-4, CT-1, CT-2, DC-1, DC-4, FL-1, MD-1, MI-3, MO-1, NY-2, NY-7, NC-1, OH-2, PA-3, WV-1, CAN-3

INTERNATIONAL JOURNAL OF AGING AND HUMAN DEVELOPMENT — CA-4, CT-1, CT-2, DC-1, DC-4, DC-6, IL-1, MD-1, MD-2, MN-1, NY-7, OH-1, OH-5, PA-3, PA-6, RI-1, PR-1, CAN-3, CAN-4, CAN-5

JOURNAL OF AGING AND SOCIAL POLICY — AZ-1, CA-4, CA-5, DC-1, DC-4, MD-1, MI-3, OH-1, OR-1, PA-3, PA-6, TN-1, WV-1

JOURNAL OF THE AMERICAN GERIATRICS SOCIETY - CA-4, CT-1, CT-2, DC-1, DC-4, FL-2, HI-1, MD-1, MD-2, MI-2, MN-1, NY-1, NY-5, NY-7, NC-1, OH-1, OH-2, PA-2, PA-3, PA-5, PA-6, WA-2, PR-1, CAN-3, CAN-4, CAN-5

JOURNAL OF CROSS-CULTURAL GERONTOLOGY — CA-3, CA-4, CT-1, DC-1, DC-4, HI-1, MD-1, MD-2, OH-2, PA-3, CAN-3, CAN-5

JOURNALS OF GERONTOLOGY — AZ-1, CA-2, CA-4, CA-5, CT-1, CT-2, DE-1, DC-1, DC-4, DC-6, FL-1, FL-2, HI-1, IL-1, MD-1, MD-2, MA-1, MA-2, MA-3, MI-1, MI-2, MI-3, MI-4, MN-1, MO-1, NE-1, NY-1, NY-4, NY-5, NY-6, NY-7, NC-1, OH-1, OH-2, OH-3, OH-4, OH-5, OR-1, PA-2, PA-3, PA-4, PA-5, PA-6, VA-1, WA-1, WA-2, PR-1, CAN-1, CAN-2, CAN-3, CAN-4, CAN-5

MECHANISMS OF AGEING AND DEVELOPMENT — CA-4, CT-1, MD-1

NEUROBIOLOGY OF AGING — CA-4, CT-1, HI-1, MD-1, PA-3

OLDER AMERICANS REPORT — AZ-1, CA-2, CA-3, CA-4, CT-2, DE-1, DC-1, DC-2, DC-4, DC-5, FL-1, FL-2, HI-1, IL-1, MD-1, MA-1, MA-3, MI-1, MI-2, MI-3, MI-4, MI-5, NY-1, NY-4, NY-6, OH-1, OH-3, OH-5, PA-2, PA-3, PA-4, PA-5, RI-1, TN-1, TX-1, WA-1, WA-2, WV-1

PROVIDER — AZ-1, CA-3, CT-2, DC-1, DC-4, MN-1, NY-7, OH-1, OH-5, PA-1, PA-3, VA-1, CAN-3

PSYCHOLOGY AND AGING — CA-4, CT-1, DC-1, FL-2, MD-1, OH-1, OH-2, PA-3, PA-6, CAN-1, CAN-2, CAN-3, CAN-4, CAN-5

RESEARCH ON AGING — CA-4, CT-1, CT-2, DC-1, DC-4, DC-6, FL-1, IL-1, MD-1, MD-2, MA-1, MN-1, MO-1, NY-6, NY-7, OH-1, PA-2, PA-3, PA-4, PA-6, TN-1, WA-2, WV-1, PR-1, CAN-1, CAN-3, CAN-4

Appendix D

Collection Strengths

ADMINISTRATION, INCLUDING NURSING HOMES, RETIREMENT FACILITIES, ETC.

AZ-1, CT-2, DC-3, DC-4, FL-1, HI-1, KS-1, MD-1, MD-2, MI-1, MI-3, MI-5, MN-1, MO-1, NY-7, NC-1, OH-1, OH-3, OH-4, OH-5, PA-1, PA-3, PA-4, TX-1, TX-2, VA-1, WV-1, CAN-2, CAN-3, CAN-4, CAN-5

AGING NETWORK REPORTS, DOCUMENTS, ETC.

AZ-1, CA-4, CA-5, DE-1, DC-1, FL-2, HI-1, KS-1, KY-1, MD-1, MI-1, MI-4, NY-2, NY-6, OH-1, OH-3, OH-5, PA-1, PA-2, PA-4, PA-5, TN-1, TX-1, VA-1, CAN-1

ANTHROPOLOGY, ETHNICITY, CROSS-CULTURAL STUDIES, ETC.

CA-3, DC-1, FL-2, HI-1, MD-1, MO-1, OH-2, PA-3, TX-2, WA-1, CAN-5

CAREGIVING, SOCIAL SERVICES, FAMILY ISSUES, ETC.

AZ-1, CA-1, CA-4, CA-5, CT-1, CT-2, DC-1, DC-4, FL-2, FL-4, HI-1, IL-1, KS-1, MA-1, MA-3, MI-2, MI-4, MI-5, MN-1, MO-1, NE-1, NY-1, NY-4, NY-5, NY-6, NY-7, OH-1, OH-2, OH-3, OH-4, OH-5, OR-1, PA-2, PA-3, PA-4, PA-6, RI-1, TN-1, TX-2, WA-1, WA-2, WV-1, PR-1, CAN-3, CAN-5

CONSUMER MATERIALS, INCLUDING EASY-TO-READ, LARGE-PRINT, ETC.

CA-1, MI-3, OH-4, TX-1

DEMOGRAPHIC, CENSUS, STATISTICAL DATA, ETC.

AZ-1, CA-2, CA-3, CA-5, DC-1, DC-5, DC-6, FL-1, FL-2, FL-3, HI-1, IL-1, IL-2, KS-1, MD-1, MD-2, MA-2, MA-3, MI-4, NY-2, NY-6, NC-1, OH-1, OH-3, OH-5, OR-1, PA-2, PA-3, PA-4, PA-5, TN-1, TX-3, WA-1, WV-1, CAN-1

DYING, DEATH, BEREAVEMENT

AZ-1, CA-1, CA-4, DC-4, FL-1, FL-3, HI-1, IL-2, NE-1, NY-1, NY-5, OH-2, OH-3, PA-3, TX-2, PR-1, CAN-4

EDUCATION, PROGRAM DEVELOPMENT, PLANNING, ETC.

AZ-1, CA-5, DE-1, FL-2, KY-1, NY-3, OR-1, TN-1

EMPLOYMENT

AZ-1, CT-2, DC-1, DC-4, MD-1, NY-6, OH-3, PA-2

GOVERNMENT PUBLICATIONS

AZ-1, CA-3, CA-4, CA-5, DE-1, DC-1, DC-3, DC-5, FL-3, HI-1, IL-1, MA-3, MI-3, MI-4, MI-5, NY-2, NY-6, NC-1, OH-3, PA-4, PA-5, TX-1, VA-1, WA-1, CAN-1, CAN-3

HEALTH CARE, HEALTH PROMOTION, ETC.

AZ-1, CA-1, CA-3, CA-5, CT-1, CT-2, DE-1, DC-1, DC-2, DC-3, DC-4, FL-1, FL-2, HI-1, MD-1, MA-1, MA-3, MI-1, MI-3, MN-1, MO-1, NY-2, NY-4, NY-5, NY-6, NY-7, NC-1, OH-2, OH-3, OH-4, OR-1, PA-1, PA-2, PA-3, PA-4, RI-1, TX-2, PR-1, CAN-1, CAN-2, CAN-3, CAN-4

HOUSING, LIVING ARRANGEMENTS, ENVIRONMENT AND PRODUCT DESIGN, ETC.

AZ-1, CA-1, CA-3, CA-4, CA-5, CT-2, DC-1, DC-4, DC-5, HI-1, IL-1, KS-1, MD-1, MA-1, MI-1, MI-2, MI-4, MO-1, NY-1, NY-5, NY-6, OH-1, OH-3, OH-4,

PA-2, PA-3, RI-1, TX-2, PR-1, CAN-1

INTERNATIONAL MATERIALS

DC-1, HI-1, OH-3, PA-3

LONG-TERM CARE

AZ-1, CA-1, CA-5, CT-1, CT-2, DC-1, DC-4, FL-4, HI-1, KS-1, MD-1, MA-1, MA-3, MI-1, MI-2, MN-1, MO-1, NY-2, NY-4, NY-5, NY-6, NY-7, NC-1, OH-1, OH-3, OH-5, OR-1, PA-1, PA-2, PA-3, PA-4, TN-1, TX-2, TX-3, VA-1, WA-2, CAN-1, CAN-2, CAN-3, CAN-4, CAN-5

MEDICARE/MEDICAID, INSURANCE, SOCIAL SECURITY, LEGAL, FINANCIAL, ETC.

AZ-1, CA-2, CA-3, CA-5, DE-1, DC-1, DC-3, DC-4, DC-5, DC-6, FL-3, HI-1, IL-1, IL-2, MD-1, MD-2, MA-1, MA-3, MI-1, MI-4, MI-5, MO-1, NY-2, NY-6, NC-1, OH-3, PA-2, PA-3, PA-4, PA-5, RI-1, TX-3, VA-1, WA-2, WV-1

MEDICINE, NURSING, REHABILITATION, ETC.

CA-1, CT-1, CT-2, DC-4, FL-1, FL-2, FL-3, HI-1, KY-1, MD-1, MA-2, MN-1, NY-1, NY-2, NY-5, NY-7, NC-1, NC-2, OH-1, OH-2, OH-4, OR-1, PA-2, PA-3, PA-4, TX-2, TX-3, WA-2, PR-1, CAN-2, CAN-3, CAN-4, CAN-5

PHYSIOLOGY, AGING PROCESS, MOLECULAR BIOLOGY, ETC.

CT-1, DE-1, FL-2, HI-1, MD-1, MA-2, NY-5, OH-3, PA-1, CAN-4

POLICY ISSUES

AZ-1, CA-3, CA-4, CA-5, CT-1, CT-2, DC-1, DC-3, DC-4, DC-5, DC-6, HI-1, IL-1, MD-2, MA-3, MI-3, MI-5, MO-1, NY-6, NC-1, OH-1, OH-3, OH-5, PA-2, PA-3, PA-5, TN-1, WA-1, WA-2, WV-1

PSYCHOLOGY, MENTAL HEALTH, COUNSELING, ETC.

CA-1, CA-4, DC-1, FL-2, FL-4, HI-1, IL-2, MD-1, MA-1, MN-1, NE-1, NY-1, NY-5, OH-1, OH-3, OR-1, PA-1, PA-2, PA-3, PA-6, CAN-4, CAN-5

RESEARCH AND STATISTICAL METHODS, ETC.

CA-5, DC-6, FL-1, FL-2, HI-1, MD-1, MA-2, MI-4, NY-2, NY-5, OH-1, PA-3, PA-4, PR-1

RETIREMENT

AZ-1, CA-1, CA-4, CT-2, DC-1, DC-4, DC-6, FL-1, IL-2, MD-1, MD-2, MA-1, MO-1, NY-6, OH-3, RI-1

Appendix E

Hardware and Software Used

(Specific software is reported below exactly as given by each respondent. Most of the integrated library systems are listed only under each specific application. In some cases it was not clear if a "shared system" was a library system or a general office system.)

HARDWARE

Microcomputers — AZ-1, CA-4, CA-5, CT-1, DC-1, DC-5, DC-6, FL-2, FL-4, HI-1, MD-1, MD-2, MA-2, MA-3, MI-2, MN-1, NE-1, NY-1, NY-7, NC-1, OH-1, OH-3, OH-4, OR-1, PA-3, PA-6, TN-1, TX-2, VA-1, WA-1, PR-1, CAN-1, CAN-3, CAN-4, CAN-5
Minicomputers — CA-1, CT-2, DC-1, DC-2, DC-4, MD-2, MN-1, OH-2
Mainframes — CA-5, MD-1, NC-1
CD-ROM — FL-2, MD-1, PA-6, CAN-3

DATABASE VENDORS USED

BRS — AZ-1, CA-2, CA-4, CT-1, CT-2, DC-1, FL-2, KY-1, MD-1, MD-2, MA-2, MI-2, MN-1, MO-1, NY-5, NC-1, OH-1, OH-4, OR-1, PA-2, PA-3, PA-4, CAN-3, CAN-4, CAN-5
CompuServe — DC-1, FL-2, MD-2, NY-7
DIALOG — CA-2, CA-4, CT-2, DC-1, DC-5, FL-4, MD-1, MD-2, MI-2, MN-1, NY-5, OH-1, PA-4, CAN-1, CAN-4
Dow Jones News/Retrieval — DC-1
LegiSlate — DC-1
Mead Data Central — DC-1, DC-6
MEDLARS — CA-5, CT-1, CT-2, MD-1, MA-2, MO-1, NY-2, NY-5, NY-7, NC-1, OH-1, OR-1, PA-3, CAN-4
PaperChase — FL-2
STN International— MD-1
USCInfo — CA-4
VU/TEXT — DC-1
Washington Alert — DC-5
Westlaw — DC-1
H. W. Wilson Company — MD-2
shared system — DC-2

SOFTWARE — SHARED SYSTEMS

Integrated Library Systems
Geac — CA-4
Melvyl — CA-5

General Systems — CT-2, DC-1, DC-2, DC-4, DC-6, MA-2, NC-1, PA-2, TX-2

SOFTWARE — APPLICATIONS

Acquisitions
B&T Link — PA-3
DataEase — OR-1
OCLC — MD-2
STAR — DC-1
Sydney — CAN-4
shared system — DC-6

AV Management
Media Minder — TX-2

Bibliographic Management
ProCite — CA-4, CT-1, CT-2, DC-1, FL-2, MD-1, NC-1, PA-3
SciMate — CT-2

Catalog (Online)
Innopac — FL-2
LUIS — FL-4
Marcon — AZ-1
OCLC — CT-2
PALS — MN-1
STAR — DC-1
Sydney — CAN-4
Winnebago — OH-3
shared system — DC-2, DC-6, MA-2, TX-2

Cataloging
DataEase — OR-1
INMAGIC — CAN-3
Librarian's Helper — PA-3

MARCIVE — NY-5
Marcon — AZ-1
OCLC — CA-4, CT-2, DC-1, FL-2, MD-1, MD-2, MN-1
ProCite — MI-2, OH-1
RLIN — CA-4
STAR — DC-1
Sydney — CAN-4
Winnebago — OH-3
shared system — DC-6, MA-2, TX-2

Circulation
DataEase — OR-1
Innopac — FL-2
OCLC — MD-2
STAR — DC-1
Sydney — CAN-4
Winnebago — OH-3
shared system — TX-2

Database Management
DBase — AZ-1, FL-2, FL-4, MD-1, MN-1, CAN-4

Desktop Publishing
Ventura — CT-2

Interlibrary Loan
DOCLINE — CT-2, MN-1, NY-7, PA-3
MINITEX — MN-1
OCLC — CA-4, DC-1, MD-2, NY-7, TX-2
RLIN — CA-4
shared system — MA-2

Serials Management
DBase — PA-3

EBSCO — NY-5
Marcon — AZ-1
REMO — CT-2, MD-1
Sydney — CAN-4
shared system — DC-1

Spreadsheet
Lotus — FL-2, MA-2, CAN-4

Word Processing
Appleworks — MN-1
Microsoft Word — FL-4, MI-2, NC-1
PFS Write — MN-1
RWord — DC-6
WordPerfect — AZ -1, CA-4, CT-2, FL-2, MD-1, MA-1, MA-2, OH-1, OH-3, CAN-3, CAN-4
Wordstar — CA-4, MA-2, PA-3
WPS Write — MA-3
shared system — DC-1, DC-2, PA-2

Bibliography

Abortion issue puts veto threat on FY'92 funding for AoA, HHS. (1991, June 21). *Older Americans Report*, 15, 242.

Achenbaum, W. Andrew. (1983). *Shades of gray: Old age, American values, and federal policies since 1920.* Boston: Little, Brown.

Achenbaum, W. Andrew. (1987). Reconstructing GSA's history. *Gerontologist*, 27, 21-29.

Adler, Marjorie. (1958). History of Gerontological Society, Inc. *Journal of Gerontology*, 13, 94-102.

Aging and long-term care: A directory of selected information resources. (1980). (Contract No. HHS 105-79-3010). (DHHS Publication No. [OHDS] 81-20304). Washington, D. C.: National Clearinghouse on Aging.

American Hospital Association. (1990). *Survey of health sciences libraries in hospitals: 1989. Survey questionnaire.* Chicago: American Hospital Association.

American Hospital Association. (1991). *Survey of health sciences libraries in hospitals: 1989. Executive summary.* Chicago: American Hospital Association.

Applications due June 28 for AoA eldercare institutes. (1991, April 26). *Older Americans Report*, 15, 161-162.

Applied Management Sciences, and Cuadra Associates. (1980). *Catalog of human services information resource organizations: An exploratory study of human services information clearing-*

houses (Contract No. HEW 100-79-0183). (Human Services Monograph Series, No. 15). Rockville, Md.: Project SHARE.

Applied Management Sciences, and Cuadra Associates. (1981). *Descriptive analysis of human services information clearinghouses* (Contract No. DHEW-100-79-0183). Rockville, Md.: Project SHARE. (NTIS No. PB81-169997)

Ardito, Stephanie C. and Marta L. Dosa. (1983). Gerontological information. In Allen Kent (Ed.), *Encyclopedia of library and information science* (Vol. 36, Supplement 1, pp. 187-219). New York: Marcel Dekker.

Bagnell, Prisca von Dorotka (Ed.). (1982). Gerontology and geriatrics collections (Special issue). *Special Collections*, 1(3/4).

Baker, Carol A., and Richard L. Bale. (1981). Anatomy of clearinghouses: Understanding how they work could lead to wiser funding. *American Society for Information Science Bulletin*, 7(3), 21-23.

BMDP data manager: 1990 software release and data manager manual. (1990). Los Angeles: BMDP Statistical Software.

Brandon, Alfred N. and Dorothy R. Hill (1991). Selected list of books and journals for the small medical library. *Bulletin of the Medical Library Association*, 79, 195-222.

Brazil, Mary Jo. (1990). *Building library collections on aging: A selection guide and core list.* Santa Barbara, Calif.: ABC-CLIO.

Brindle, Elizabeth A., Marta L. Dosa, and Gerald M. Gee. (1977). A prototype gerontological information program. In American Society for Information Science, *Information management in the 1980s: Proceedings of the 40th ASIS Annual Meeting, Chicago, Illinois* (Vol. 14, p. 7-abstract and microfiche text). White Plains, N.Y.: Knowledge Industry Publications.

Butler, Robert N. (1987). National Institute on Aging. In George L. Maddox (Ed.), *The encyclopedia of aging* (pp. 468-470). New York: Springer.

Catalogs of the Ethel Percy Andrus Gerontology Center, University of Southern California, Los Angeles. (1976). (Vols. 1-2). Boston: G. K. Hall.

Corcoran, Virginia H. (1982, November). *Information for service providers: What is the impact*. Discussion session, 35th Annual Scientific Meeting of the Gerontological Society of America. Boston.

Cowdry, Edmund Vincent. (Ed.). (1939). *Problems of ageing: Biological and medical aspects*. Baltimore: Williams & Wilkins.

Craig, Bruce M. (1982). Weighing the issues and consequences of federal program termination: Administration on Aging support for career preparation. *Gerontology and Geriatrics Education*, 3, 129-137.

Darnay, Brigitte T., and Janice A. DeMaggio. (Eds.). (1990). *Directory of Special Libraries and Information Centers* (13th ed.). Detroit: Gale Research.

Democrats plan new strategy for OAA programs. (1981, June 17). *Older American Reports*, 5(24), 1-2.

Dosa, Marta L. (1978). The gerontological information program. *American Society for Information Science Bulletin*, 5(1), 18.

Dosa, Marta L., and Elizabeth A. Brindle. (1979, November). *Impact of information and data support for practitioners working with the elderly*. Paper presented at the 32nd Annual Scientific Meeting of the Gerontological Society, Washington, DC.

Dresser, Peter D., and Karen Hill. (Eds.). (1990). *Research Centers Directory* (14th ed.). Detroit: Gale Research.

Duwors, Elaine, Joanne Gard Marshall, and Gale Moore. (1982). Canadian information resources and services in gerontology and geriatrics. *Special Collections*, 1(3/4), 119-129.

Ficke, Susan Coombs. (Ed.). (1985). *An orientation to the Older Americans Act* (Revised ed.). Washington, D.C.: National Association of State Units on Aging.

First SCAN contract awarded. (1978). *Aging*, Nos. 287-288, 47.

Gelfand, Donald E. (1988). *The aging network: Programs and services* (3rd ed.). New York: Springer.

Geriatric education centers. (1989). Washington, D.C.: Department of Health and Human Services, Public Health Service, Health Resources and Services Administration.

Gilbert, Alice. (1981, November). *Gerontological resources: Tapping into the information connection.* Discussion session, 34th Annual Scientific Meeting of the Gerontological Society of America. Toronto, Ontario.

Grant, Madeline. (1986). The best little library on aging in Canada. *Canadian Library Journal*, 43, 57-58.

A guide to selected information resources in aging. (1980). (Contract No. HHS 105-79-3010). (DHHS Publication No. [OHDS] 81-20303). Washington, D.C.: National Clearinghouse on Aging.

Halpin, Peter. (1985). Transferring a national information system from the public sector to the private sector: How the Administration on Aging did it. *Journal of the American Society for Information Science*, 36, 53-55.

Hernon, Peter, and Charles R. McClure. (1987). *Federal information policies in the 1980s: Conflicts and issues*. Norwood, N.J.: Ablex, 1987,

Hesslein, Shirley B. (1986). *Serials on aging: An analytical guide.* New York: Greenwood.

Hickey, Tom. (1978). Association for Gerontology in Higher Education: A brief history. In Mildred M. Seltzer, Harvey Sterns, and Tom Hickey (Eds.), *Gerontology in higher education: Perspectives and issues* (pp. 2-11). Belmont, Calif.: Wadsworth.

House Republican move could cost OAA millions. (1981, July 8). *Older American Reports*, 5(27), 3-4.

Hubbard, Richard W., and Jerome Kowal. (Eds.). (1988). Geriatric education centers (Special issue). *Gerontology and Geriatrics Education*, 8(3/4).

Jacobs, Bruce. (1990). Aging and politics. In Robert H. Binstock and Linda K. George (Eds.), *Handbook of aging and the social sciences* (3rd ed.) (pp. 349-361). San Diego: Academic Press.

Kemper, Peter, and Randall S. Brown. (1986). *The evaluation of the National Long Term Care Demonstration: Final report* (Rev. ed.) (Contract No. HHS-100-80-0157). Princeton, N.J.: Mathematica Policy Research.

Larson, Signe, and Mary Jane Ruhl. (1981). Cuts hit information community. *American Society for Information Science Bulletin*, 7(4), 10.

Longo, Margaret Kronauer, Stewart R. Greathouse, and Jean E. Mueller. (1982). Integrating information technology in gerontology: The Andrus Gerontological Information Center. *Special Collections*, 1(3/4), 27-42.

Lovas, Paula M. (1982). The National Gerontology Resource Center: The public perspective. *Special Collections*, 1(3/4), 43-52.

Miller, Emily H., and Neal E. Cutler. (1976). Toward a comprehensive information system in gerontology: A survey of problems, resources, and potential solutions. *Gerontologist*, 16, 198-206.

New National Aging Resource Centers. (1989). *Philadelphia Corporation for Aging Update*, 89(4), 1, 5, 7.

Oriol, William E. (1987). Information and the "aging network." In Karen B. Levitan (Ed.), *Government infostructures: A guide to the network of information resources and technologies at federal, state, and local levels* (pp.173-185). New York: Greenwood.

Owens, H. Jean. (1978). An analytical survey of libraries in gerontological centers. *Educational Gerontology*, 3, 345-353.

Owens, H. Jean. (1980). *Directory of gerontological libraries and information centers*. Detroit: Wayne State University-University of Michigan, Institute of Gerontology.

Peterson, David A., and Elizabeth B. Douglass. (1990). The impact of Administration on Aging funding on gerontology instruction. *Journal of Aging & Social Policy*, 2(3/4), 169-182.

Rafferty, Eve. (1982). Guidelines for the selection and acquisition of gerontological materials. *Behavioral & Social Sciences Librarian*, 2(2/3), 39-56.

Rafferty, Eve. (1983, April). *Networking among gerontological and geriatric resource centers: Summary of a survey*. Paper presented at the 29th annual meeting of the Western Gerontological Society, Albuquerque, New Mexico. (ERIC Document Reproduction Service, ED 237-104)

Rafferty, Eve, and Marta L. Dosa. (1980, November). *Information resources for the aging and for gerontology: Implications for the White House Conference on Aging*. Discussion session, 33rd Annual Scientific Meeting of the Gerontological Society of America. San Diego, California.

Reagan deferrals could mean big loss to senior centers. (1981, February 25). *Older American Reports*, 5(8), 5.

Reagan signs rescissions bill, AAA funds restored. (1981, June 10). *Older American Reports*, 5(23), 1-2.

Shock, Nathan W. (1951). *A classified bibliography of gerontology and geriatrics*. Stanford, Calif.: Stanford University Press.

Shock, Nathan W. (1957). *A classified bibliography of gerontology and geriatrics: Supplement one 1949-1955*. Stanford, Calif.: Stanford University Press.

Shock, Nathan W. (1963). *A classified bibliography of gerontology and geriatrics: Supplement two 1956-1961*. Stanford, Calif.: Stanford University Press.

Shock, Nathan W. (1982). Historical perspectives: United States. In Willie M. Edwards and Frances Flynn (Eds.), *Gerontology: A cross-national core list of significant works* (pp. 27-39). Ann Arbor: University of Michigan, Institute of Gerontology.

Shock, Nathan W. (1987). Baltimore Longitudinal Study of Aging. In George L. Maddox (Ed.), *The encyclopedia of aging* (pp. 52-54). New York: Springer.

Shock, Nathan W., Marta L. Dosa, Margaret E. Monroe, Willie Edwards, and Frances Flynn. (1977, November). *A review of the Classified Bibliography of Gerontology and Geriatrics and Current Publications in Gerontology and Geriatrics*. Discussion session, 30th Annual Scientific Meeting of the Gerontological Society, San Francisco.

Shock, Nathan W., Richard C. Greulich, Reubin Andres, David Arenberg, Paul T. Costa, Jr., Edward G. Lakatta, and Jordan D. Tobin. (1984). *Normal human aging: The Baltimore Longitudinal Study of Aging* (NIH Publication No. 84-2450). Washington D.C.: U. S. Government Printing Office.

Simson, Sharon, and Laura Bleiweiss Wilson. (1981). The performance of Administration on Aging multidisciplinary gerontology centers for education and training. *Educational Gerontology*, 7, 215-229.

Smith, Donald. (1983). The National Clearinghouse on Aging. *Behavioral & Social Sciences Librarian*, 3(2), 19-30.

Subject index to the SCAN microfiche collection. (1987). (Vols. 1-2). Washington, D.C.: American Association of Retired Persons.

Thesaurus of aging terminology: AgeLine database on middle age and aging. (1991). (4th ed.). Washington, D.C.: American Association of Retired Persons.

United States. Administration on Aging. National Clearinghouse on Aging. (1975). *Thesaurus*. Los Angeles: Documentation Associates Information Services.

United States. Administration on Aging. National Clearinghouse on Aging. (1977). *Thesaurus* (2d ed.). (DHEW Publication No. [OHDS] 78-20087). Los Angeles: Documentation Associates Information Services.

United States. Congress. Office of Technology Assessment. (1990). *Confused minds, burdened families: Finding help for people with Alzheimer's and other dementias* (OTA-BA-403). Washington, D.C.: U.S. Government Printing Office.

United States. Congress. Senate. Special Committee on Aging. (1974). *Developments in Aging: 1973 and January-March 1974* (Senate Report 93-846). Washington, D.C.: U.S. Government Printing Office.

United States. Congress. Senate. Special Committee on Aging. (1975). *Developments in Aging: 1974 and January-April 1975* (Senate Report 94-250). Washington, D.C.: U.S. Government Printing Office.

United States. Congress. Senate. Special Committee on Aging. (1976). *Developments in Aging: 1975 and January-May 1976: Part 2. Appendixes* (Senate Report 94-998). Washington, D.C.: U.S. Government Printing Office.

United States. Congress. Senate. Special Committee on Aging. (1977). *Developments in Aging: 1976: Part 2. Appendixes* (Senate Report 95-88). Washington, D.C.: U.S. Government Printing Office.

United States. Congress. Senate. Special Committee on Aging. (1978). *Developments in Aging: 1977: Part 2. Appendixes* (Senate Report 95-771). Washington, D.C.: U.S. Government Printing Office.

United States. Congress. Senate. Special Committee on Aging. (1979). *Developments in Aging: 1978: Part 2. Appendixes* (Senate Report 96-66). Washington, D.C.: U.S. Government Printing Office.

United States. Congress. Senate. Special Committee on Aging. (1980). *Developments in Aging: 1979: Part 2. Appendixes* (Senate Report 96-613). Washington, D.C.: U.S. Government Printing Office.

United States. Congress. Senate. Special Committee on Aging. (1981). *Developments in Aging: 1980: Part 2. Appendixes* (Senate Report 97-62). Washington, D.C.: U.S. Government Printing Office.

United States. Congress. Senate. Special Committee on Aging. (1982). *Developments in Aging: 1981: Vol. 1. Appendix* (Senate Report 97-314). Washington, D.C.: U.S. Government Printing Office.

United States. Congress. Senate. Special Committee on Aging. (1991). *Developments in Aging: 1990: Vol. 2. Appendixes*. (Senate Report 102-28). Washington, D.C.: U.S. Government Printing Office.

United States. Executive Office of the President. Office of Management and Budget. (1981, September 11). *Memorandum to the heads of executive departments and agencies. Subject: Federal information centers* (M-81-14). Washington, D.C.

United States. General Accounting Office. (1976). *Conditions of older people: National information system needed* (GAO Report No. HRD 79-95). Washington, D.C.: U.S. Government Printing

Index

(Boldface numbers in library/collection name entries refer to their full descriptions in the directory part of this book.)

About the Author

JOYCE A. POST is the Librarian of the Philadelphia Geriatric Center. She has extensive experience as a librarian and research consultant, has written several books and articles for professional journals, and has compiled several bibliographies and indexes. Her publications include *Travel in the United States: A Guide to Information Sources* (1982) and *TV Guide 25 Year Index, by Author and Subjects* (1979).